ZERO TO FINALS

Obstetrics and Gynaecology

First Edition 2020
ISBN: 9798603797267

Dr Thomas Watchman
MbChB (hons) BSc (Psychology) MSc (Medical Education) MRCGP MRCP (UK) DCH FHEA
General Practitioner (GP)
Manchester, United Kingdom

Copyright Zero to Finals 2020. All rights reserved.

No part of this book can be reproduced or transmitted in any way without prior permission from Dr Thomas Watchman at Zero to Finals. Email: tom@zerotofinals.com.

About Zero to Finals

My name is Tom. I started Zero to Finals in 2016 to build the resource I wish I had during medical school. As you may imagine for someone that creates educational resources, I love learning and teaching. So much so I completed a psychology degree and a degree in medical education to find ways I could get better at both. After graduating, I felt the need to keep learning, for my own knowledge and to have the tools to teach others. I kept studying and taking exams, achieving the MRCP (UK) Diploma from the Royal College of Physicians and the Diploma in Child Health (DCH) from the Royal College of Paediatrics and Child Health. I completed my GP training in August 2020, and started working as a GP.

I always dreamed of creating a resource that focuses on helping medical students achieve more in medical school and eases the burden of facing complicated and overwhelming textbooks, lectures and journals. I took a year out of training after the UK foundation program with the objective of making this dream a reality. I have been working on it non-stop ever since. I love creating books, notes, questions, illustrations, podcasts and videos to help students in any way I can.

The Zero to Finals books are designed to be studied from cover to cover in preparation for your exams. I have removed the waffle and focused on the key information that is tested in exams. I do my best to cover all the big topics as well as the smaller details that will help you avoid knowledge gaps. The focus is on learning the concepts, vocabulary and latest guidelines so you can take the fastest route to exam success and proficiency as a new doctor. I have added *TOM TIP*s, which are pearls of wisdom I have gained over more than a decade of sitting medical exams.

The Zero to Finals books are supplemented by the resources on the website. If you struggle to follow the notes in this book or to get your head around a topic, head over to zerotofinals.com. There is a webpage on each topic with illustrations, diagrams, podcasts and videos that tackle the problem from every angle.

To get in touch or report an error please email me at tom@zerotofinals.com.

Disclaimer

It is important that you use Zero to Finals for its intended purpose: as a resource to help students and health professionals prepare for exams. It is not intended and should not be used as a resource, guideline or reference for clinical practice or decision making. It is certainly not designed for patients looking for medical information or advice. There are plenty of very good resources for the above, not least your senior colleagues, guidelines, research papers or personal doctor. By using the Zero to Finals resources you agree that Zero to Finals and those involved in creating the resources are not responsible for any actions you take or don't take based on the information provided.

The skills needed to practice medicine, paediatrics and other healthcare roles are broad and complex. There is a limit to what you can learn from one resource. You need to develop clinical judgment, experience and context specific decision making skills that cannot be learned in one place. It is important to develop your own ability to find the best resources and data to make decisions about your clinical practice. Attend clinical placements, listen to your tutors and supervisors, ask for help and use a variety of up to date guidelines, protocols, research and other resources when preparing for exams and treating patients. Nothing is completely reliable and accurate.

I employ extensive effort to ensure the information is accurate and up to date, however it is not perfect, and research, guidelines and best practice are always changing. There will be errors despite my best efforts. I would be very grateful if you point them out when you find them, so I can correct them. Don't accept anything as fact without questioning it.

For Carolyn

A marvellous role model, mentor and listener
Thank you for helping me become a GP

CONTENTS

1	The Reproductive System	5
2	Gynaecology	20
3	Cancer	70
4	Genitourinary Medicine	82
5	Contraception	103
6	Fertility	124
7	Early Pregnancy	134
8	Antenatal Care	146
9	Labour and Delivery	191
10	Postnatal Care	222

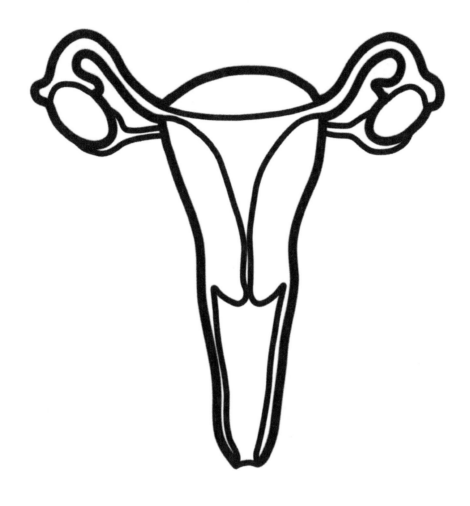

THE REPRODUCTIVE SYSTEM

1.1	Female Sex Hormones	6
1.2	Female Puberty	6
1.3	The Menstrual Cycle	7
1.4	Ovulation, Conception and Implantation	9
1.5	Development of the Embryo	12
1.6	Development of the Placenta	12
1.7	Function of the Placenta	14
1.8	Physiological Changes in Pregnancy	15
1.9	Labour and Delivery	18

Female Sex Hormones

The female sex hormones are the basis of the **menstrual cycle**, **conception**, **pregnancy**, **contraception**, **menopause** and **hormone replacement therapy**. It is worth spending time becoming familiar and comfortable with these hormones, as this will make learning everything else in obstetrics and gynaecology much easier.

Hypothalamic–Pituitary–Gonadal Axis

The hypothalamus releases **gonadotropin-releasing hormone** (**GnRH**). GnRH stimulates the **anterior pituitary** to produce **luteinising hormone** (**LH**) and **follicle-stimulating hormone** (**FSH**).

LH and FSH stimulate the development of **follicles** in the **ovaries**. The **theca granulosa cells** around the follicles secrete **oestrogen**. **Oestrogen** has a **negative feedback** effect on the **hypothalamus** and **anterior pituitary** to suppress the release of **GnRH**, **LH** and **FSH**.

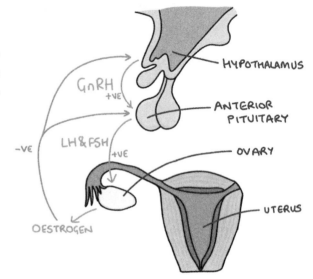

Oestrogen

Oestrogen is a **steroid sex hormone** produced by the ovaries in response to **LH** and **FSH**. The most prevalent and active version is **17-beta oestradiol**. It acts on tissues with **oestrogen receptors** to promote **female secondary sexual characteristics**. It stimulates:
- Breast tissue development
- Growth and development of the female sex organs (vulva, vagina and uterus) at puberty
- Blood vessel development in the uterus
- Development of the endometrium

Progesterone

Progesterone is a **steroid sex hormone** produced by the **corpus luteum** after **ovulation**. When pregnancy occurs, progesterone is produced mainly by the **placenta** from 10 weeks gestation onwards. Progesterone acts on tissues that have previously been stimulated by **oestrogen**. Progesterone acts to:
- Thicken and maintain the endometrium
- Thicken the cervical mucus
- Increase the body temperature

Female Puberty

In childhood, girls have relatively little **GnRH**, **LH**, **FSH**, **oestrogen** and **progesterone** in their system. During puberty, these hormones start to increase sequentially, causing the development of **female secondary sexual characteristics**, the onset of the **menstrual cycle** and the ability to conceive children.

Puberty starts age **8 - 14 in girls** and **9 - 15 in boys**. It takes about **four years** from start to finish. Girls have their pubertal growth spurt earlier in puberty than boys.

Overweight children tend to enter puberty at an earlier age. **Aromatase** is an **enzyme** found in **adipose** (fat) tissue, that is important in the creation of **oestrogen**. Therefore, the more **adipose tissue** present, the higher the quantity of the enzyme responsible for oestrogen creation. There may be **delayed puberty** in girls with low birth weight, chronic disease or eating disorders, and in athletes.

In girls, puberty starts with the development of **breast buds**, followed by **pubic hair** and finally the onset of **menstrual periods**. The first episode of menstruation is called **menarche**. Menstrual periods usually begin about two years from the start of puberty.

Tanner Staging

The stage of pubertal development can be determined using the **Tanner scale**, based on examination findings of secondary sexual characteristics.

Tanner Stage	Age	Pubic Hair	Breast Development
Stage I	Under 10	No pubic hair	No breast development
Stage II	10 - 11	Light and thin	Breast buds form behind the areola
Stage III	11 - 13	Course and curly	Breast begins to elevate beyond the areola
Stage IV	13 - 14	Adult like but not reaching the thigh	Areolar mounds form and project from surrounding breast
Stage V	Above 14	Hair extending to the medial thigh	Areolar mounds reduce, and adult breasts form

Hormonal Changes During Puberty

Growth hormone (**GH**) increases initially, causing a spurt in growth during the initial phases of puberty.

The **hypothalamus** starts to secrete **GnRH**, initially during sleep, then throughout the day in the later stages of puberty. GnRH stimulates the release of **FSH** and **LH** from the **pituitary gland**. FSH and LH stimulate the ovaries to produce **oestrogen** and **progesterone**. FSH levels **plateau** about a year before menarche. LH levels continue to rise, and spike just before they induce menarche.

Oestrogen suppresses **growth hormone**, causing growth to slow down as oestrogen levels increase. This suppression is the reason the growth spurt finishes sooner in girls, leaving them shorter than boys going into adulthood.

The Menstrual Cycle

The menstrual cycle consists of two phases: the **follicular phase** and the **luteal phase**. The **follicular phase** is from the start of **menstruation** to the moment of **ovulation** (the first 14 days in a 28-day cycle). The **luteal phase** is from the moment of **ovulation** to the start of **menstruation** (the final 14 days of the cycle).

The Follicular Phase

From puberty, the ovaries have a finite number of cells that have the potential to develop into eggs. These cells are called **oocytes**. **Granulosa cells** surround the oocytes, forming structures called **follicles**.

Follicles go through four key stages of development in the ovaries:
- **Primordial follicles**
- **Primary follicles**
- **Secondary follicles**
- **Antral follicles** (also known as **Graafian follicles**)

The process of **primordial follicles** maturing into **primary** and **secondary follicles** is always occurring, independent of the menstrual cycle. Once the follicles reach the **secondary follicle** stage, they have the receptors for **follicle stimulating hormone (FSH)**. Further development after the **secondary follicle** stage requires stimulation from **FSH**.

At the start of the menstrual cycle, **FSH** stimulates further development of the **secondary follicles**. As the follicles grow, the **granulosa cells** that surround them secrete increasing amounts of **oestradiol** (oestrogen). The oestradiol has a **negative feedback** effect on the **pituitary gland**, reducing the quantity of **LH** and **FSH** produced. The rising **oestrogen** also causes the **cervical mucus** to become more permeable, allowing sperm to penetrate the cervix around the time of **ovulation**.

One of the follicles will develop further than the others and become the **dominant follicle**. **Luteinising hormone (LH)** spikes just before ovulation, causing the **dominant follicle** to release the **ovum** (an **unfertilised egg**) from the ovary. **Ovulation** happens 14 days before the end of the menstrual cycle, for example, day 14 of a 28-day cycle, or day 16 of a 30-day cycle.

The Luteal Phase

After ovulation, the **follicle** that released the **ovum** collapses and becomes the **corpus luteum**. The **corpus luteum** secretes high levels of **progesterone**, which maintains the **endometrial lining**. This **progesterone** also causes the **cervical mucus** to become thick and no longer penetrable. The corpus luteum also secretes a small amount of **oestrogen**.

When fertilisation occurs, the **syncytiotrophoblast** of the **embryo** secretes **human chorionic gonadotropin (HCG)**. HCG **maintains** the **corpus luteum.** Without hCG, the corpus luteum degenerates. Pregnancy tests check for **hCG** to confirm a pregnancy.

When there is no fertilisation of the ovum, and no production of **hCG**, the **corpus luteum** degenerates and stops producing oestrogen and progesterone. This fall in oestrogen and progesterone causes the **endometrium** to break down and **menstruation** to occur. Additionally, the **stromal cells** of the **endometrium** release **prostaglandins**. Prostaglandins encourage the endometrium to break down and the uterus to contract. **Menstruation** starts on **day 1** of the menstrual cycle. The **negative feedback** from oestrogen and progesterone on the **hypothalamus** and **pituitary gland** ceases, allowing the levels of **LH** and **FSH** to begin to rise, and the cycle to restart.

Menstruation

Menstruation involves the superficial and middle layers of the **endometrium** separating from the basal layer. The tissue is broken down inside the **uterus**, and released via the cervix and vagina. The release of fluid containing blood from the vagina lasts 1 - 8 days.

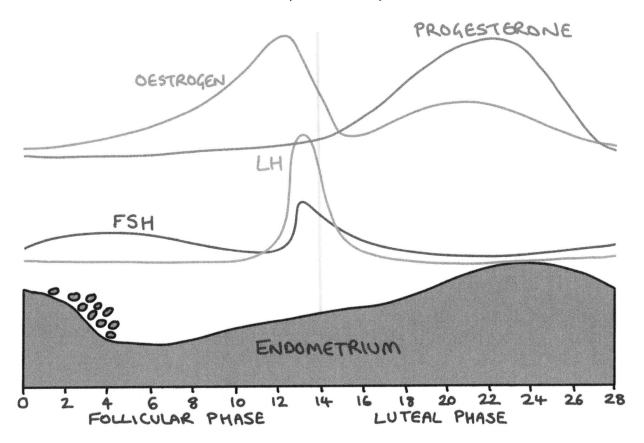

Ovulation, Conception and Implantation

Primordial follicles each contain a ***primary oocyte***. The ***oocytes*** are the ***germ cells*** (first generation of sex cell) that eventually undergo ***meiosis*** to become the ***mature ovum***, ready for ***fertilisation***. They contain the full **46 chromosomes**. These ***primordial follicles*** and ***oocytes*** spend the majority of their lives in a resting state inside the ***ovaries***, waiting for their time to develop. The ***primary oocyte*** is contained within the ***pregranulosa cells***, surrounded by the outer ***basal lamina layer***.

Development of the Primary Follicle

Primordial follicles grow and become ***primary follicles***. These ***primary follicles*** have three layers:
- The ***primary oocyte*** in the centre
- The ***zona pellucida***
- The cuboidal shaped ***granulosa*** cells

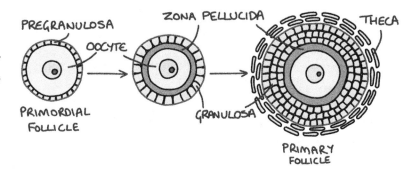

The ***granulosa cells*** secrete the material that becomes the ***zona pellucida***. They also secrete ***oestrogen***.

As the ***follicles*** grow larger, they develop a further surrounding layer called the ***theca folliculi***. The inner layer of the ***theca folliculi*** is called the ***theca interna***. The theca interna secretes ***androgen*** hormones. The outer layer, called the ***theca externa***, is made up of ***connective tissue*** cells containing ***smooth muscle*** and ***collagen***.

Development of the Secondary Follicle

The process of **primordial follicles** maturing into **primary** and **secondary follicles** is always occurring, independent of the menstrual cycle. As **primary follicles** become **secondary follicles**, they grow larger and develop small fluid-filled gaps between the granulosa cells. Once the follicles reach the **secondary follicle** stage, they have receptors for **follicle stimulating hormone** (**FSH**). Further development after the **secondary follicle** stage requires stimulation from **FSH**. At the start of the menstrual cycle, **FSH** stimulates further development of the **secondary follicles**.

Development of the Antral Follicles

With further development, the **secondary follicle** develops a single large fluid-filled area within the granulosa cells called the **antrum**. **Antrum** refers to a natural chamber within a structure. This is the **antral follicle** stage. This antrum fills with increasing amounts of fluid, making the follicle expand rapidly. The **corona radiata** is made of granulosa cells, and surrounds the **zona pellucida** and the **oocyte**.

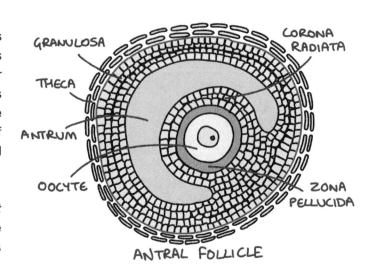

At this point, one of the follicles becomes the **dominant follicle**. The other follicles start to degrade, while the dominant follicle grows to become a mature follicle. This follicle bulges through the wall of the ovary.

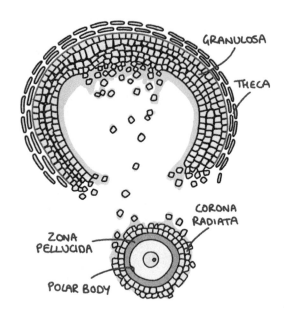

Ovulation

When there is a surge of **luteinising hormone** (**LH**) from the pituitary, it causes the smooth muscle of the **theca externa** to squeeze, and the follicle to burst. Follicular cells also release digestive enzymes that puncture a hole in the wall of the ovary, allowing the ovum to escape. The oocyte is released into the area surrounding the ovary. At this point, it is floating in the peritoneal cavity, but it is quickly swept up by the **fimbriae** of the **fallopian tubes**.

Corpus Luteum

The leftover parts of the follicle collapse and turn a yellow colour. The collapsed follicle becomes the **corpus luteum**. The cells of the granulosa and theca interna become **luteal cells**. Luteal cells secrete steroid hormones, most notably **progesterone**. The corpus luteum persists in response to **human chorionic gonadotropin** (**HCG**) from a fertilised **blastocyst** when pregnancy occurs. When fertilisation does not occur, the corpus luteum degenerates after 10 to 14 days.

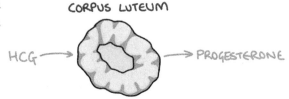

Fertilisation

Just before and around the time of ovulation, the **primary oocyte** undergoes **meiosis**. This process splits the full **46 chromosomes** in the oocyte (a **diploid** cell) into two, leaving only **23 chromosomes** (a **haploid** cell). The other 23 chromosomes float off to the side and become something called a **polar body**. It is then a **secondary oocyte**.

The Reproductive System

The female egg (ovum) at this stage still has the surrounding layers from its time in the follicle. In the middle is the oocyte with the first polar body, surrounded by the *zona pellucida* and the granulosa cells that make up the *corona radiata*.

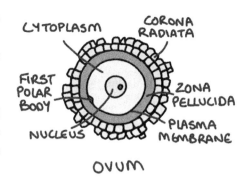

When sperm from the male enter the fallopian tube via the vagina and uterus, they will attempt to penetrate the *corona radiata* and *zona pellucida* to fertilise the egg. Usually, only one sperm will get through before the surrounding layers shut the other sperm out.

When a sperm enters the egg, the 23 chromosomes of the egg multiply into two sets. One set of 23 chromosomes combine with the 23 chromosomes from the sperm to form a diploid set of 46 chromosomes, and the other set of 23 chromosomes float off to the side and create the *second polar body*.

Development of the Blastocyst

The combination of the 23 chromosomes from the egg and 23 chromosomes from the sperm combine to form a fertilised cell called a *zygote*. This cell divides rapidly to create a mass of cells called the *morula*. During this process, the mass of cells travels along the fallopian tube toward the uterus.

While travelling, a fluid-filled cavity gathers within the group of cells, and it becomes a *blastocyst*. The blastocyst contains the main group of cells in the middle, called the *embryoblast*. Alongside the *embryoblast* is a fluid-filled cavity called the *blastocele*. Surrounding the embryoblast and the blastocele is an outer layer of cells called the *trophoblast*. At this point, it gradually loses the *corona radiata* and *zona pellucida*. When the *blastocyst* enters the uterus, it contains 100 - 150 cells.

Implantation

When the *blastocyst* arrives at the uterus, 8 - 10 days after *ovulation*, it reaches the endometrium. The cells of the trophoblast (the outer layer of the blastocyst) undergo *adhesion* to the stroma (supportive outer tissue) of the *endometrium*. The outer layer of the trophoblast is called the syncytiotrophoblast. This layer forms projections into the stroma. The cells of the syncytiotrophoblast mix with the cells of the endometrium.

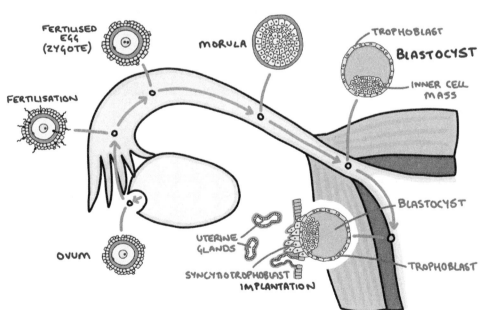

The cells of the *stroma* convert into a tissue called *decidua* that is specialised in providing nutrients to the *trophoblast*. When the *blastocyst* implants on the *endometrium*, the *syncytiotrophoblast* starts to produce **human chorionic gonadotropin** (**HCG**). HCG is very important for maintaining the *corpus luteum* in the ovary, allowing it to continue producing *progesterone* and *oestrogen*.

Development of the Embryo

A week after fertilisation, the implanted **blastocyst** starts to differentiate into various types of cell. The cells of the **embryoblast** split in two, with the **yolk sac** on one side and the **amniotic cavity** on the other. The **embryonic disc** sits between the **yolk sac** and the **amniotic cavity**. The cells of the embryonic disc develop into the **fetal pole**, and eventually into the fetus.

The **chorion** surrounds this complex. The **chorion** has two layers: the **cytotrophoblast** and the **syncytiotrophoblast**. The **cytotrophoblast** is the inner layer and the **syncytiotrophoblast** is the outer layer, which is embedded in the endometrium.

Basic Embryology

Over a short time, a space called the **chorionic cavity** forms around the **yolk sac**, **embryonic disc** and **amniotic sac**. These structures are suspended from the chorion by the **connecting stalk**, which will eventually become the umbilical cord.

At around five weeks gestation, the **embryonic disc** develops into a **fetal pole** containing three layers: the **ectoderm** (outer layer), **mesoderm** (middle layer) and **endoderm** (inner layer). These three layers go on to become all the different tissues of the body.

The **ectoderm** becomes the:
- GI tract
- Lungs
- Liver
- Pancreas
- Thyroid
- Reproductive system

The **mesoderm** becomes the:
- Heart
- Muscles
- Bone
- Connective tissue
- Blood
- Kidneys

The **ectoderm** becomes the:
- Skin
- Hair
- Nails
- Teeth
- Central nervous system

At around six weeks gestation, the **fetal heart** forms and starts to beat. The **spinal cord** and **muscles** also begin to develop. The embryo (**fetal pole**) is about 4mm in length.

At around eight weeks gestation, all the major organs have started to develop. From this point onwards the fetus matures and grows until birth.

Development of the Placenta

During the **follicular phase** of the menstrual cycle, the **endometrium** thickens and gets ready for a fertilised egg to arrive. The **myometrium** sends off **artery branches** into the endometrium. Initially, these arteries grow straight outwards like plant shoots. As they continue to grow, they coil into a spiral. These thick-walled and coiled arteries are bunched together, making the endometrial tissue highly vascular. These are known as the **spiral arteries**.

Placental and Umbilical Cord Development

When the **blastocyst** implants on the **endometrium**, the outermost layer, called the **syncytiotrophoblast**, grows into the **endometrium**. It forms finger-like projections called **chorionic villi**. The chorionic villi contain fetal blood vessels.

The chorionic villi nearest the connecting stalk of the developing embryo are the most vascular and contain **mesoderm**. This area is called the **chorion frondosum**. The cells in the **chorion frondosum** proliferate and become the placenta. The **connecting stalk** becomes the **umbilical cord**. Placental development is usually complete by 10 weeks gestation.

Development of the Lacunae

Trophoblast invasion of the endometrium sends signals to the **spiral arteries** in that area, reducing their **vascular resistance** and making them more fragile. The blood flow to these arteries increases, and eventually they break down, leaving pools of blood called **lacunae** (lakes). Maternal blood flows from the **uterine arteries**, into these **lacunae**, and back out through the **uterine veins**. *Lacunae* form at around 20 weeks gestation.

These **lacunae** surround the **chorionic villi**, separated by the **placental membrane**. Oxygen, carbon dioxide and other substances can diffuse across the **placental membrane** between the maternal and fetal blood.

When the process of forming lacunae is inadequate, the woman can develop **pre-eclampsia**. Pre-eclampsia is caused by high **vascular resistance** in the **spiral arteries**. High vascular resistance in the spiral arteries results in a sharp rise in maternal blood pressure, and leads to a number of complications in the mother and fetus.

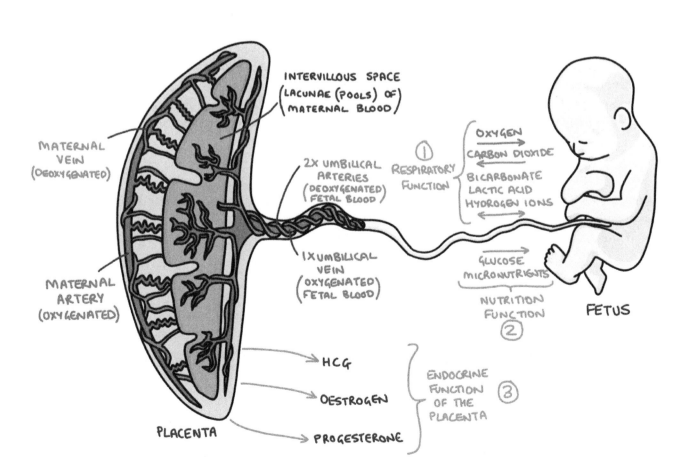

Function of the Placenta

Respiration

The placenta is the only source of **oxygen** for the fetus. **Fetal haemoglobin** has a higher **affinity** for oxygen than **adult haemoglobin**. The fetal haemoglobin is more attractive to oxygen molecules than the maternal haemoglobin. As a result, when maternal blood and fetal blood are nearby in the placenta, oxygen is drawn off the maternal haemoglobin, across the placental membrane, onto the fetal haemoglobin. **Carbon dioxide**, **hydrogen ions**, **bicarbonate** and **lactic acid** are also exchanged in the placenta, allowing the fetus to maintain a healthy **acid-base balance**.

Nutrition

All of the nutrition for the fetus comes from the mother. This nutrition is mostly in the form of glucose, which is used for energy and growth. The placenta can also transfer vitamins and minerals to the fetus, as well as potentially harmful substances if the mother is consuming medications, alcohol, caffeine or cigarette smoke.

Excretion

The placenta performs a similar function to kidneys in a child or adult, filtering waste products from the fetus. These waste products include **urea** and **creatinine**.

Endocrine

Human Chorionic Gonadotropin

The **syncytiotrophoblast** produces **hCG**. HCG levels increase in early pregnancy, plateau at around ten weeks gestation, then start to fall. HCG helps to maintain the **corpus luteum** until the placenta can take over the production of **oestrogen** and **progesterone**. HCG can cause symptoms of nausea and vomiting in early pregnancy. Higher levels of hCG occur with **multiple pregnancy** (e.g. twins) and **molar pregnancy**. **Pregnancy tests** look for hCG as a marker of pregnancy.

Oestrogen

The placenta produces **oestrogen**, which helps to soften tissues and make them more flexible. Oestrogen allows the muscles and ligaments of the uterus and pelvis to expand, and the cervix to become soft and ready for birth. It also enlarges and prepares the breasts and nipples for breastfeeding.

Progesterone

The placenta mostly takes over the production of **progesterone** by five weeks gestation. The role of progesterone is to maintain the pregnancy. It causes relaxation of the uterine muscles (preventing contraction and labour) and maintains the endometrium. It causes side effects by relaxing other muscles, such as the **lower oesophageal sphincter** (causing heartburn), the **bowel** (causing constipation) and the **blood vessels** (causing hypotension, headaches and skin flushing). It also raises the body temperature between 0.5 and 1 degree Celsius.

Immunity

The mother's **antibodies** can transfer across the placenta to the fetus during pregnancy. These antibodies allow the fetus to benefit from the long term immunity of the mother during the pregnancy and shortly after birth. An example of this is with **recurrent genital herpes**, where the mother's antibodies to the herpes virus cross the placenta and protect the baby during labour and delivery, preventing infection during birth. This protection does not occur during an initial episode of genital herpes, as the mother has not yet started producing sufficient antibodies against the herpes virus to offer the fetus protection.

Physiological Changes in Pregnancy

The body goes through a large number of changes during pregnancy. You will come across pregnant women with a high heart rate, low blood pressure, abnormal blood test results and skin changes. It helps to know what changes are normal in healthy pregnant women and when to investigate further for underlying disease.

Hormonal Changes

The **anterior pituitary gland** produces more **ACTH**, **prolactin** and **melanocyte stimulating hormone** in pregnancy.

Higher **ACTH** levels cause a rise in **steroid hormones**, particularly **cortisol** and **aldosterone**. Higher steroid levels lead to an improvement in most autoimmune conditions and a susceptibility to diabetes and infections.

Increased prolactin acts to suppress **FSH** and **LH**, causing reduced **FSH** and **LH** levels.

Increased **melanocyte stimulating hormone** causes increased **pigmentation** of the skin during pregnancy, resulting in skin changes such as **linea nigra** and **melasma**.

TSH remains normal, but **T3** and **T4** levels rise.

HCG levels rise, roughly doubling every 48 hours until they plateau around 8 - 12 weeks, then gradually start to fall.

Progesterone levels rise throughout pregnancy. Progesterone acts to maintain the pregnancy, prevent contractions and suppress the mother's immune reaction to **fetal antigens**. The **corpus luteum** produces progesterone until ten weeks gestation. The placenta produces it during the remainder of the pregnancy.

Oestrogen rises throughout pregnancy, produced by the **placenta**.

Changes to the Uterus, Cervix and Vagina

The size of the **uterus** increases from around 100g to 1.1kg during pregnancy. There is **hypertrophy** of the **myometrium** and the **blood vessels** in the uterus. Increased oestrogen may cause **cervical ectropion** and increased **cervical discharge**. Oestrogen also causes **hypertrophy** of the **vaginal muscles** and increased **vaginal discharge**. The changes in the vagina prepare it for delivery, however they make **bacterial** and **candidal infection** (thrush) more common.

Before delivery, **prostaglandins** break down **collagen** in the **cervix**, allowing it to **dilate** and **efface** during childbirth.

Cardiovascular Changes

There are several cardiovascular changes during pregnancy:
- Increased **blood volume**
- Increased **plasma volume**

- Increased **cardiac output**, with increased **stroke volume** and **heart rate**
- Decreased **peripheral vascular resistance**
- Decreased **blood pressure** in early and middle pregnancy, returning to normal by term
- **Varicose veins** can occur due to peripheral vasodilation and obstruction of the inferior vena cava by the uterus
- **Peripheral vasodilation** also causes flushing and hot sweats

Respiratory Changes

Tidal volume and *respiratory rate* increase in later pregnancy, to meet the increased oxygen demands.

Renal Changes

A number of changes in the kidneys happen during pregnancy:
- Increased **blood flow** to the kidneys
- Increased **glomerular filtration rate** (**GFR**)
- Increased **aldosterone** leads to increased salt and water reabsorption and retention
- Increased **protein excretion** from the kidneys (normal is up to 0.3g in 24 hours)
- Dilatation of the **ureters** and **collecting system**, leading to a **physiological hydronephrosis** (more right-sided)

Haematology and Biochemistry Changes

There is increased **red blood cell production** in pregnancy, leading to higher **iron**, **folate** and **B12** requirements. **Plasma volume** increases **more** than **red blood cell volume**, leading to a lower **concentration** of **red blood cells**. High plasma volume means the **haemoglobin concentration** and **red cell concentration** (**haematocrit**) fall in pregnancy, resulting in **anaemia**.

Clotting factors such as **fibrinogen** and **factor VII**, **VIII** and **X** increase in pregnancy, making women **hyper-coagulable**. This increases the risk of **venous thromboembolism** (blood clots developing in the veins). Pregnant women are more likely to develop **deep vein thrombosis** and **pulmonary embolism**.

There are a few other changes you may find on blood results:
- Increased **white blood cells**
- Decreased **platelet count**
- Increased **ESR** and **D-dimer**
- Increased **alkaline phosphatase** (**ALP**), up to 4 times normal, due to secretion by the **placenta**
- Reduced **albumin** due to loss of proteins in the kidneys
- **Calcium** requirements increase, but so does gut absorption of calcium, meaning calcium levels remain stable

Skin and Hair Changes

Several changes to skin are normal in pregnancy:
- Increased **skin pigmentation** due to increased **melanocyte stimulating hormone**, with **linea nigra** and **melasma**
- **Striae gravidarum** (stretch marks on the expanding abdomen)
- General itchiness (**pruritus**) can be normal, but can indicate **obstetric cholestasis**
- **Spider naevi**
- **Palmar erythema**

Postpartum hair loss is normal, and usually improves within six months.

The Reproductive System

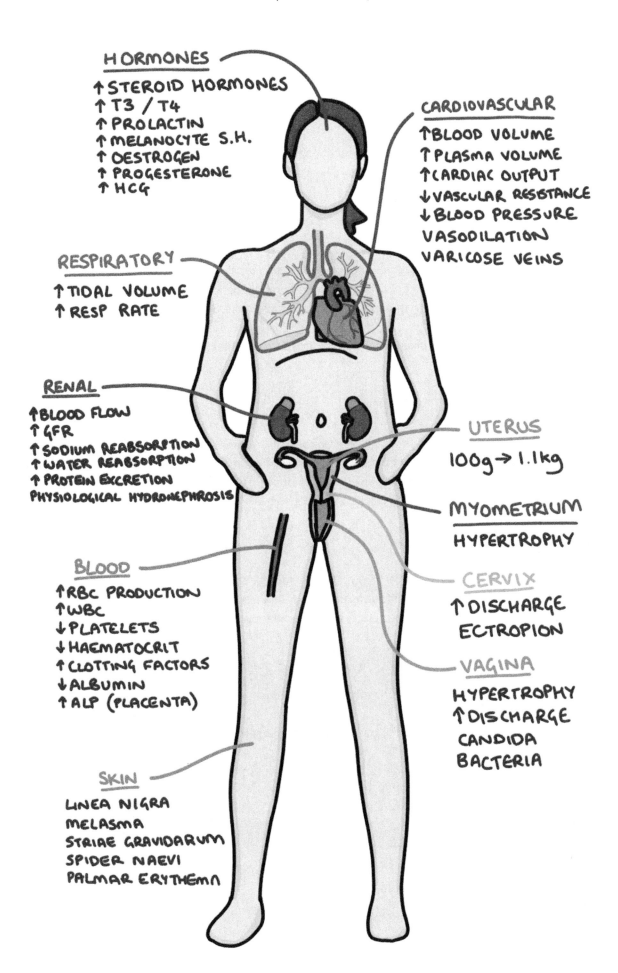

Labour and Delivery

Labour and delivery normally occur between 37 and 42 weeks gestation.

There are three stages of labour:
- **The first stage** is from the onset of labour (true contractions) until 10cm cervical dilatation
- **The second stage** is from 10cm cervical dilatation to delivery of the baby
- **The third stage** is from delivery of the baby to delivery of the placenta

Prostaglandins

Prostaglandins act like local hormones, triggering specific effects in local tissues. Tissues throughout the entire body contain and respond to prostaglandins. They play a crucial role in menstruation and labour by stimulating contraction of the uterine muscles. They also have a role in the ripening of the cervix before delivery.

One key prostaglandin to be aware of is **prostaglandin E2**. **Pessaries** containing prostaglandin E2 (**dinoprostone**) can be used to **induce** labour.

Braxton-Hicks Contractions

Braxton-Hicks contractions are occasional irregular contractions of the uterus. They are usually felt during the second and third trimester. Women can experience temporary and irregular tightening or mild cramping in the abdomen. These are not true contractions, and they do not indicate the onset of labour. They do not progress or become regular. Staying hydrated and relaxing can help reduce Braxton-Hicks contractions.

First Stage

The first stage of labour is from the onset of labour (true contractions) until the cervix is fully dilated to 10cm. It involves **cervical dilation** (opening up) and **effacement** (getting thinner). The "**show**" refers to the **mucus plug** in the cervix that prevents bacteria from entering the uterus during pregnancy, falling out and creating space for the baby to pass through.

The first stage has three **phases**:
- **Latent phase**: From 0 to 3cm dilation of the cervix. This progresses at around 0.5cm per hour. There are irregular contractions.
- **Active phase**: From 3cm to 7cm dilation of the cervix. This progresses at around 1cm per hour, and there are regular contractions.
- **Transition phase**: From 7cm to 10cm dilation of the cervix. This progresses at around 1cm per hour, and there are strong and regular contractions.

Second Stage

The second stage of labour lasts from 10cm dilatation of the cervix to delivery of the baby. The success of the second stage depends on "**the three Ps**": **power**, **passenger** and **passage**.

Power: the strength of the uterine contractions.

Passenger: the four descriptive qualities of the fetus:
- **Size**: particularly the size of the head as this is the largest part.
- **Attitude**: the posture of the fetus. For example, how the back is rounded and how the head and limbs are flexed.
- **Lie**: the position of the fetus in relation to the mother's body:
  - Longitudinal lie - the fetus is straight up and down.
  - Transverse lie - the fetus is straight side to side.
  - Oblique lie - the fetus is at an angle.
- **Presentation**: the part of the fetus closest to the cervix:
  - Cephalic presentation - the head is first.
  - Shoulder presentation - the shoulder is first.
  - Breech presentation - the legs are first. This can be:
    - Complete breech - with hips and knees flexed (like doing a cannonball jump into a pool)
    - Frank breech - with hips flexed and knees extended, bottom first
    - Footling breech - with a foot hanging through the cervix

Passage: the size and shape of the passageway, mainly the pelvis.

Cardinal Movements of Labour

There are seven cardinal movements of labour:
- **Engagement**: the top of the baby's head enters the pelvic inlet in a transverse (side-to-side) position
- **Descent**: the baby's head descends past the pelvic inlet into the pelvic cavity
- **Flexion**: the baby's head flexes chin to chest, presenting the narrowest area of the head
- **Internal rotation**: the baby's head rotates so the sagittal suture is in an anterior-posterior (front-to-back) position
- **Extension**: the head passes through the pelvic outlet, the head extends and the head is born
- **Restitution and external rotation**: the head rotates to a transverse position so the shoulders match the pelvic outlet
- **Expulsion**: the anterior shoulder, then the posterior shoulder, then the rest of the body are born

Descent

Obstetricians describe the position of the baby's head in relation to the mother's *ischial spines* during the descent phase. Descent is measured in centimetres, from:
- **-5**: when the baby is high up at around the pelvic inlet
- **0**: when the head is at the ischial spines (this is when the head is "*engaged*")
- **+5**: when the fetal head has descended further out

Third Stage

The third stage of labour is from the completed birth of the baby to the delivery of the placenta.

Physiological management is where the placenta is delivered by maternal effort without medications or cord traction.

Active management of the third stage is where the midwife or doctor assist in delivery of the placenta. Active management shortens the third stage and reduces the risk of bleeding. **Haemorrhage**, or more than a **60-minute delay** in delivery of the placenta, should prompt **active management**. Active management can be associated with **nausea** and **vomiting**.

Active management involves giving a dose of **intramuscular oxytocin** to help the uterus contract and expel the placenta. Careful traction is applied to the **umbilical cord** to guide the placenta out of the uterus and vagina.

GYNAECOLOGY

2.1	Differential Diagnosis in Gynaecology	21
2.2	Primary Amenorrhoea	23
2.3	Secondary Amenorrhoea	26
2.4	Premenstrual Syndrome	27
2.5	Heavy Menstrual Bleeding	29
2.6	Fibroids	31
2.7	Endometriosis	33
2.8	Adenomyosis	36
2.9	Menopause	37
2.10	Premature Ovarian Insufficiency	39
2.11	Hormone Replacement Therapy	40
2.12	Polycystic Ovarian Syndrome	46
2.13	Ovarian Cysts	50
2.14	Ovarian Torsion	53
2.15	Asherman's Syndrome	54
2.16	Cervical Ectropion	55
2.17	Nabothian Cysts	56
2.18	Pelvic Organ Prolapse	57
2.19	Urinary Incontinence	59
2.20	Atrophic Vaginitis	63
2.21	Bartholin's Cyst	64
2.22	Lichen Sclerosus	64
2.23	Female Genital Mutilation	66
2.24	Congenital Structural Abnormalities	67
2.25	Androgen Insensitivity Syndrome	69

Differential Diagnosis in Gynaecology

There are a limited number of presenting complaints in gynaecology. Having a list of **differential diagnoses** in your head when a patient presents with **intermenstrual bleeding** or **pelvic pain** can help you take a focused history and perform a relevant examination to narrow down that list of differentials. This will make you appear practiced and knowledgeable in OSCE examinations, and help make it easier when seeing patients in real life. Some causes are responsible for many presenting complaints, and while the lists initially appear intimidating, as you learn about the core conditions in gynaecology, they will become easier to remember.

Amenorrhoea

Amenorrhoea refers to a lack of menstrual periods. The causes of amenorrhoea is a big topic and covered in more detail later on.

Primary amenorrhoea is when the patient has never developed periods. This can be due to:
- Abnormal functioning of the hypothalamus or pituitary gland (**hypogonadotropic hypogonadism**)
- Abnormal functioning of the gonads (**hypergonadotropic hypogonadism**)
- Imperforate hymen or other structural pathology

Secondary amenorrhoea is when the patient previously had periods that subsequently stopped. This can be due to:
- Pregnancy (the most common cause)
- Menopause
- Physiological stress due to excessive exercise, low body weight, chronic disease or psychosocial factors
- Polycystic ovarian syndrome
- Medications, such as hormonal contraceptives
- Premature ovarian insufficiency (menopause before 40 years)
- Thyroid hormone abnormalities (hyper or hypothyroid)
- Excessive prolactin, from a prolactinoma
- Cushing's syndrome

Irregular Menstruation

Abnormal uterine bleeding refers to irregularities in the **menstrual cycle**, affecting frequency, duration, regularity of the cycle length and the volume of menses. Irregular menstrual periods indicate **anovulation** (a lack of ovulation) or irregular ovulation. This occurs due to disruption of the normal hormonal levels in the menstrual cycle, or ovarian pathology. It can be due to:
- Extremes of reproductive age (early periods or perimenopause)
- Polycystic ovarian syndrome
- Physiological stress (excessive exercise, low body weight, chronic disease and psychosocial factors)
- Medications, particularly progesterone only contraception, antidepressants and antipsychotics
- Hormonal imbalances, such as thyroid abnormalities, Cushing's syndrome and high prolactin

Intermenstrual Bleeding

Intermenstrual bleeding (**IMB**) refers to any bleeding that occurs between menstrual periods. This is a **red flag** that should make you consider cervical and other cancers, although other causes are more common.

The key causes of *intermenstrual bleeding* are:

- Hormonal contraception
- Cervical ectropion, polyps or cancer
- Sexually transmitted infection
- Endometrial polyps or cancer
- Vaginal pathology, including cancers
- Pregnancy
- Ovulation can cause spotting in some women
- Medications, such as SSRIs and anticoagulants

Dysmenorrhoea

Dysmenorrhoea describes painful periods. The causes are:

- Primary dysmenorrhoea (no underlying pathology)
- Endometriosis or adenomyosis
- Fibroids
- Pelvic inflammatory disease
- Copper coil
- Cervical or ovarian cancer

Heavy Menstrual Periods

Menorrhagia refers to heavy menstrual bleeding. This can be caused by:

- **Dysfunctional uterine bleeding** (no identifiable cause)
- Extremes of reproductive age
- Fibroids
- Endometriosis and adenomyosis
- Pelvic inflammatory disease (infection)
- Contraceptives, particularly the copper coil
- Anticoagulant medications
- Bleeding disorders (e.g. **Von Willebrand disease**)
- Endocrine disorders (diabetes and hypothyroidism)
- Connective tissue disorders
- Endometrial hyperplasia or cancer
- Polycystic ovarian syndrome

Postcoital Bleeding

Postcoital bleeding (**PCB**) refers to bleeding after sexual intercourse. This is a **red flag** that should make you consider cervical and other cancers, although other causes are more common. Often **no cause** is found. The key causes are:

- Cervical cancer, ectropion or infection
- Trauma
- Atrophic vaginitis
- Polyps
- Endometrial cancer
- Vaginal cancer

Pelvic Pain

Pelvic pain can be acute or chronic. The presentation of pelvic pain varies significantly. A detailed history and examination are usually able to identify the cause. There are a large number of possible causes, including:

- Urinary tract infection
- Dysmenorrhoea (painful periods)
- Irritable bowel syndrome (IBS)
- Ovarian cysts
- Endometriosis
- Pelvic inflammatory disease (infection)
- Ectopic pregnancy
- Appendicitis
- Mittelschmerz (cyclical pain during ovulation)
- Pelvic adhesions
- Ovarian torsion
- Inflammatory bowel disease (IBD)

Vaginal Discharge

Vaginal discharge is a normal physiological finding. Excessive, discoloured or foul-smelling discharge may indicate:

- Bacterial vaginosis
- Candidiasis (thrush)
- Chlamydia
- Gonorrhoea
- Trichomonas vaginalis
- Foreign body
- Cervical ectropion
- Polyps
- Malignancy
- Pregnancy
- Ovulation (cyclical)
- Hormonal contraception

Pruritus Vulvae

Pruritus vulvae refers to *itching* (pruritus) of the *vulva* and *vagina*. There are a large number of causes:
- *Irritants* such as soaps, detergents and barrier contraception
- *Atrophic vaginitis*
- *Infections* such as *candidiasis* (thrush) and pubic lice
- Skin conditions such as eczema
- Vulval malignancy
- Pregnancy-related vaginal discharge
- Urinary or faecal incontinence
- Stress

Primary Amenorrhoea

Primary amenorrhoea is defined as not starting menstruation:
- By 13 years when there is no other evidence of pubertal development
- By 15 years of age where there are other signs of puberty, such as breast bud development

Normal Puberty

Puberty starts age 8 - 14 in girls and 9 - 15 in boys. It takes about four years from start to finish. Girls have their **pubertal growth spurt** earlier in puberty than boys. In girls, puberty starts with the development of **breast buds**, then **pubic hair**, and finally **menstrual periods** about two years from the start of puberty.

Hypogonadism

Hypogonadism refers to a lack of the **sex hormones**, **oestrogen** and **testosterone**, that normally rise before and during puberty. A lack of these hormones cause a delay in puberty. The lack of sex hormones is fundamentally due to one of two reasons:
- *Hypogonadotropic hypogonadism*: a deficiency of LH and FSH
- *Hypergonadotropic hypogonadism*: a lack of *response* to LH and FSH by the gonads (the testes and ovaries)

Hypogonadotropic Hypogonadism

Hypogonadotropic hypogonadism involves **deficiency** of **LH** and **FSH**, leading to deficiency of the sex hormones (i.e. **oestrogen**). LH and FSH are **gonadotropins** produced by the **anterior pituitary gland** in response to **gonadotropin releasing hormone** (**GnRH**) from the **hypothalamus**. Since no **gonadotropins** are simulating the **ovaries**, they do not respond by producing sex hormones (**oestrogen**). Therefore, "hypogonadotropism" causes "hypogonadism".

A deficiency of LH and FSH is the result of abnormal functioning of the **hypothalamus** or **pituitary gland**. This could be due to:
- *Hypopituitarism* (under production of pituitary hormones)
- Damage to the **hypothalamus** or **pituitary**, for example, by radiotherapy or surgery for cancer
- *Significant chronic conditions* can temporarily delay puberty (e.g. **cystic fibrosis** or **inflammatory bowel disease**)
- *Excessive exercise* or *dieting* can delay the onset of menstruation in girls
- *Constitutional delay in growth and development* is a temporary delay in growth and puberty without underlying physical pathology
- Endocrine disorders such as **growth hormone deficiency**, **hypothyroidism**, **Cushing's** or **hyperprolactinaemia**
- *Kallman syndrome*

Kallman Syndrome

Kallman syndrome is a genetic condition causing **hypogonadotrophic hypogonadism**, with failure to start puberty. It is associated with a **reduced or absent sense of smell** (*anosmia*).

Hypergonadotropic Hypogonadism

Hypergonadotropic hypogonadism is where the **gonads** fail to **respond** to stimulation from the **gonadotropins** (**LH** and **FSH**). Without negative feedback from the sex hormones (i.e. **oestrogen**), the **anterior pituitary** produces increasing amounts of **LH** and **FSH**. Consequently, you get **high gonadotropins** ("*hypergonadotropic*") and **low sex hormones** ("*hypogonadism*").

Hypergonadotropic hypogonadism is the result of abnormal functioning of the gonads. This could be due to:
- Previous damage to the **gonads** (e.g. **torsion**, **cancer** or **infections** such as **mumps**)
- Congenital absence of the ovaries
- Turner's syndrome (XO)

Congenital Adrenal Hyperplasia

Congenital adrenal hyperplasia is caused by a **congenital deficiency** of the **21-hydroxylase enzyme**. This causes **underproduction** of **cortisol** and **aldosterone**, and **overproduction** of **androgens** from birth. It is a genetic condition inherited in an **autosomal recessive** pattern. In a small number of cases, it involves a deficiency of **11-beta-hydroxylase** rather than **21-hydroxylase**.

In severe cases, the neonate is unwell shortly after birth, with **electrolyte disturbances** and **hypoglycaemia**. In mild cases, female patients can present later in childhood or at puberty with typical features:
- Tall for their age
- Facial hair
- Absent periods (primary amenorrhoea)
- Deep voice
- Early puberty

Androgen Insensitivity Syndrome

Androgen insensitivity syndrome is a condition occur in males, where the tissues are unable to respond to androgen hormones (e.g. testosterone), meaning typical male sexual characteristics do not develop. It results in a **female phenotype**, other than the internal pelvic organs. Patients have normal female external genitalia and breast tissue. Internally there are testes in the abdomen or inguinal canal, and an **absent** uterus, upper vagina, fallopian tubes and ovaries.

Structural Pathology

Structural pathology in the pelvic organs can prevent menstruation. If the ovaries are unaffected, there will be typical secondary sexual characteristics, but no menstrual periods. There may be **cyclical abdominal pain** as **menses** build up but are unable to escape through the vagina. Structural pathology that can cause primary amenorrhoea include:
- Imperforate hymen
- Transverse vaginal septae
- Vaginal agenesis
- Absent uterus
- Female genital mutilation

Assessment

Assessment aims to look for evidence of puberty and to assess for possible underlying causes. The first step is to take a detailed history of their general health, development, family history, diet and lifestyle. Examination is required to assess height, weight, stage of pubertal development and features of any underlying conditions.

The threshold for initiating investigations is **no evidence** of pubertal changes in a girl aged 13. Investigation can also be considered when there is **some evidence** of puberty but **no progression** after two years.

Initial investigations assess for underlying medical conditions:
- **Full blood count** and **ferritin** for anaemia
- **U&E** for chronic kidney disease
- **Anti-TTG** or **anti-EMA** antibodies for coeliac disease

Hormonal blood tests assess for hormonal abnormalities:
- **FSH** and **LH** will be low in hypogonadotropic hypogonadism and high in hypergonadotropic hypogonadism
- **Thyroid function tests**
- **Insulin-like growth factor I** is used as a screening test for **GH deficiency**
- **Prolactin** is raised in hyperprolactinaemia
- **Testosterone** is raised in polycystic ovarian syndrome, androgen insensitivity syndrome and congenital adrenal hyperplasia

Genetic testing with a *microarray* test to assess for underlying genetic conditions such as **Turner's syndrome** (XO).

Imaging can be useful:
- **Xray of the wrist** to assess bone age and inform a diagnosis of **constitutional delay**
- **Pelvic ultrasound** to assess the ovaries and other pelvic organs
- **MRI of the brain** to look for pituitary pathology and assess the olfactory bulbs in possible Kallman syndrome

Management

Management of primary amenorrhoea involves establishing and treating the underlying cause. Where necessary, **replacement hormones** can induce menstruation and improve symptoms. Patients with **constitutional delay in growth and development** may only require reassurance and observation.

Where the cause is due to stress or low body weight secondary to diet and exercise, treatment involves a **reduction in stress**, **cognitive behavioural therapy** and **healthy weight gain**.

Where the cause is due to an underlying chronic or endocrine condition, management involves optimising treatment for that condition.

In patients with **hypogonadotrophic hypogonadism**, such as **hypopituitarism** or **Kallman syndrome**, treatment with **pulsatile GnRH** can be used to induce ovulation and menstruation. This has the potential to induce fertility. Alternatively, where pregnancy is not wanted, **replacement sex hormones** in the form of the **combined contraceptive pill** may be used to induce regular menstruation and prevent the symptoms of oestrogen deficiency.

In patients with an ovarian cause of amenorrhoea, such as polycystic ovarian syndrome, damage to the ovaries or absence of the ovaries, the **combined contraceptive pill** may be used to induce regular menstruation and prevent the symptoms of oestrogen deficiency.

Secondary Amenorrhoea

Secondary amenorrhea is defined as no menstruation for **more than three months** after previous regular menstrual periods. Consider assessment and investigation after **three to six months**. In women with previously infrequent irregular periods, consider investigating after **six to twelve months**.

Causes

- **Pregnancy** is the most common cause
- **Menopause** and **premature ovarian failure**
- **Hormonal contraception** (e.g. IUS or POP)
- Hypothalamic or pituitary pathology
- Ovarian causes such as **polycystic ovarian syndrome**
- Uterine pathology such as **Asherman's syndrome**
- Thyroid pathology
- Hyperprolactinaemia

The **hypothalamus** reduces the production of **GnRH** in response to significant **physiological** or **psychological stress**. This leads to **hypogonadotropic hypogonadism** and amenorrhoea. The hypothalamus responds this way to prevent pregnancy in situations where the body may not be fit for it, for example:
- Excessive exercise (e.g. athletes)
- Low body weight and eating disorders
- Chronic disease
- Psychological stress

Pituitary causes of secondary amenorrhoea include:
- **Pituitary tumours**, such as a prolactin-secreting **prolactinoma**
- **Pituitary failure** due to trauma, radiotherapy, surgery or Sheehan syndrome

Hyperprolactinaemia

High prolactin levels act on the **hypothalamus** to prevent the release of **GnRH**. Without GnRH, there is no release of **LH** and **FSH**. This causes **hypogonadotropic hypogonadism**. Only 30% of women with a high prolactin level will have **galactorrhea** (breast milk production and secretion).

The most common cause of hyperprolactinaemia is a **pituitary adenoma** secreting **prolactin**. Where there are high prolactin levels, a CT or MRI scan of the brain is used to assess for a pituitary tumour. Often there is a **microadenoma** that will not appear on the initial scan, and follow up scans are required to identify tumours that may develop later.

Often no treatment is required for hyperprolactinaemia. **Dopamine agonists** such as **bromocriptine** or **cabergoline** can be used to reduce prolactin production. These medications treat **hyperprolactinaemia**, **Parkinson's disease** and **acromegaly**.

Assessment

Assessment of secondary amenorrhoea involves:
- Detailed history and examination to assess for potential causes
- Hormonal blood tests
- Ultrasound of the pelvis to diagnose **polycystic ovarian syndrome**

Hormone Tests

Beta human chorionic gonadotropin (**HCG**) urine or blood tests are required to diagnose or rule out **pregnancy**.

Luteinising hormone and **follicle-stimulating hormone**:
- High **FSH** suggests primary ovarian failure
- High **LH**, or **LH:FSH** ratio, suggests **polycystic ovarian syndrome**

Prolactin can be measured to assess for **hyperprolactinaemia**, followed by an **MRI** to identify a **pituitary tumour**.

Thyroid stimulating hormone (TSH) can screen for thyroid pathology. This is followed by **T3** and **T4** when the TSH is abnormal.
- **Raise** TSH and **low** T3 and T4 indicate **hypothyroidism**
- **Low** TSH and **raised** T3 and T4 indicate **hyperthyroidism**

Raise testosterone indicates **polycystic ovarian syndrome**, **androgen insensitivity syndrome** or **congenital adrenal hyperplasia**.

Management

Management of secondary amenorrhoea involves establishing and treating the underlying cause. Where necessary, **replacement hormones** can induce menstruation and improve symptoms.

TOM TIP: It is worth remembering that women with polycystic ovarian syndrome require a withdrawal bleed every 3 - 4 months to reduce the risk of endometrial hyperplasia and endometrial cancer. Medroxyprogesterone for 14 days, or regular use of the combined oral contraceptive pill, can be used to stimulate a withdrawal bleed.

Osteoporosis

Patients with amenorrhoea associated with low oestrogen levels are at increased risk of osteoporosis. Where the amenorrhoea lasts more than 12 months, treatment is indicated to reduce the risk of osteoporosis:
- Ensure adequate **vitamin D** and **calcium** intake
- **Hormone replacement therapy** or the **combined oral contraceptive pill**

Premenstrual Syndrome

Premenstrual syndrome (**PMS**) describes the psychological, emotional and physical symptoms that occur during the **luteal phase** of the **menstrual cycle**, particularly in the days prior to the onset of menstruation. These symptoms can be distressing and significantly impact quality of life.

Most women will experience some of the symptoms of premenstrual syndrome. The critical aspects are the severity of the symptoms, and the impact these symptoms have on the woman's functioning and quality of life.

The symptoms of PMS **resolve** once menstruation begins. Symptoms are not present **before menarche**, **during pregnancy** or **after menopause**. These are key things to note when you take a history.

Pathophysiology

Premenstrual syndrome is thought to be caused by fluctuation in **oestrogen** and **progesterone** levels during the **menstrual cycle**. The exact mechanism is not known, but it may be due to increased **sensitivity** to **progesterone** or an interaction between the sex hormones and the neurotransmitters **serotonin** and **GABA**.

Presentation

There is a long list of symptoms that can occur with premenstrual syndrome, and these will vary with the individual. Common symptoms include:

- Low mood
- Anxiety
- Mood swings
- Irritability
- Bloating
- Fatigue
- Headaches
- Breast pain
- Reduced confidence
- Cognitive impairment
- Clumsiness
- Reduced libido

These symptoms can occur in the absence of menstruation after a hysterectomy, endometrial ablation or on the Mirena coil, as the ovaries continue to function and the hormonal cycle continues. They can also occur in response to the **combined contraceptive pill** or **cyclical hormone replacement therapy** containing **progesterone**, and this is described as **progesterone-induced premenstrual disorder**.

When features are severe and have a significant effect on quality of life, this is called **premenstrual dysphoric disorder**.

Diagnosis

Diagnosis is made based on a **symptom diary** spanning two menstrual cycles. The symptom diary should demonstrate **cyclical symptoms** that occur just before, and resolve after, the onset of menstruation. A definitive diagnosis may be made, under the care of a specialist, by administering a **GnRH analogues** to halt the menstrual cycle and temporarily induce a menopause-like state, to see if the symptoms resolve.

Management

This section is based on the **RCOG Green-top guidelines** from 2016, and the **NICE CKS** updated May 2019. The following management options can be initiated in primary care:
- General healthy lifestyle changes, such as improving diet, exercise, alcohol, smoking, stress and sleep
- Combined contraceptive pill (COCP)
- SSRI antidepressants
- Cognitive behavioural therapy (CBT)

RCOG recommends COCPs containing **drospirenone** first line (i.e. **Yasmin**). Drospironone has **antimineralocortioid** effects, similar to spironolactone. **Continuous use** of the pill, as opposed to cyclical use, may be more effective.

Severe cases should be managed by a **multidisciplinary team**, involving GPs, gynaecologists, psychologists and dieticians.

Continuous transdermal oestrogen (patches) can be used to improve symptoms. **Progestogens** are required for **endometrial protection** against **endometrial hyperplasia** when using oestrogen. This can be in the form of low dose **cyclical progestogens** (e.g. norethisterone) to trigger a withdrawal bleed, or the **Mirena coil**.

Gynaecology

GnRH analogues can be used to induce a menopausal state. They are very effective at controlling symptoms; however, they are reserved for severe cases due to the adverse effects (e.g. osteoporosis). **Hormone replacement therapy** can be used to add back the hormones to mitigate these effects.

Hysterectomy and bilateral oophorectomy can be used to induce menopause where symptoms are severe and medical management has failed. **Hormone replacement therapy** will be required, particularly in women under 45 years.

Danazole and ***tamoxifen*** are options for cyclical breast pain, initiated and monitored by a breast specialist.

Spironolactone may be used to treat the physical symptoms of PMS, such as breast swelling, water retention and bloating.

Heavy Menstrual Bleeding

Heavy menstrual bleeding is also called ***menorrhagia***. On average, women lose 40 ml of blood during menstruation. Excessive menstrual blood loss involves more than 80 ml lost. The volume of blood loss is rarely measured in practice. The diagnosis is based on symptoms, such as changing pads every 1 - 2 hours, bleeding lasting more than seven days and passing large clots. A diagnosis can be made based on a self-report of "very heavy periods". Heavy menstrual periods can have a significant impact on quality of life.

Causes

- **Dysfunctional uterine bleeding** (no identifiable cause)
- Extremes of reproductive age
- Fibroids
- Endometriosis and adenomyosis
- Pelvic inflammatory disease (infection)
- Contraceptives, particularly the copper coil
- Anticoagulant medications
- Bleeding disorders (e.g. **Von Willebrand disease**)
- Endocrine disorders (diabetes and hypothyroidism)
- Connective tissue disorders
- Endometrial hyperplasia or cancer
- Polycystic ovarian syndrome

History

There are key things to ask about in any presentation with a gynaecological problem:
- Age at menarche
- Cycle length, days menstruating and variation
- Intermenstrual bleeding and post coital bleeding
- Contraceptive history
- Sexual history
- Possibility of pregnancy
- Plans for future pregnancies
- Cervical screening history
- Migraines with or without aura (for the pill)
- Past medical history and past drug history
- Smoking and alcohol history
- Family history

Investigations

Pelvic examination with a ***speculum*** and ***bimanual*** should be performed, unless there is straightforward history of heavy menstrual bleeding without other risk factors or symptoms, or they are young and not sexually active. This is mainly to assess for fibroids, ascites and cancers.

Full blood count should be performed in all women with heavy menstrual bleeding, to look for **iron deficiency anaemia**.

Outpatient hysteroscopy should be arranged if there is:
- Suspected submucosal fibroids
- Suspected endometrial pathology, such as endometrial hyperplasia or cancer
- Persistent intermenstrual bleeding

Pelvic and transvaginal ultrasound should be arranged if there is:
- Possible large fibroids (palpable pelvic mass)
- Possible adenomyosis (associated pelvic pain or tenderness on examination)
- Examination is difficult to interpret (e.g. obesity)
- Hysteroscopy is declined

Additional tests to consider in women with additional features:
- **Swabs** if there is evidence of infection (e.g. abnormal discharge or suggestive sexual history)
- **Coagulation screen** if there is a family history of clotting disorders (e.g. **Von Willebrand disease**) or periods have been heavy since menarche
- **Ferritin** if they are clinically anaemic
- **Thyroid function tests** if there are additional features of hypothyroidism

Management

Start by excluding underlying pathology such as anaemia, fibroids, bleeding disorders and cancer. Where causes are identified, these should be managed initially. For example, menorrhagia caused by a copper coil should resolve when the coil is removed. The next step is to establish whether contraception is required or acceptable.

When the woman does **not** want contraception; treatment can be used during menstruation for symptomatic relief, with:
- **Tranexamic acid** when there is no associated pain (antifibrinolytic - reduces bleeding)
- **Mefenamic acid** when there is associated pain (NSAID - reduces bleeding and pain)

Management when contraception is wanted or acceptable is with:
1. **Mirena coil** (first line)
2. **Combined oral contraceptive pill**
3. **Cyclical oral progestogens**, such as norethisterone 5mg three times daily from day 5 - 26 (although this is associated with progestogenic side effects and an increased risk of venous thromboembolism)

Progesterone only contraception may also be tried, as it can suppress menstruation. This could be a **progestogen-only pill** or a **long-acting progestogen** (e.g. depo injection or implant).

Referral to a specialist for further investigation and management is indicated if treatment is unsuccessful, symptoms are severe or there are large fibroids (more than 3 cm).

The options when medical management has failed are **endometrial ablation** and **hysterectomy.**

Endometrial ablation involves destroying the endometrium. The first generation of ablative techniques involved a hysteroscopy and direct destruction of the endometrium. This has been replaced by **second generation, non-hysteroscopic** techniques that are safer and faster. A typical example of one of these techniques involves passing a specially designed balloon into the endometrial cavity and filling it with high-temperature fluid that burns the endometrial lining. This is called **balloon thermal ablation**.

Fibroids

Fibroids are benign tumours of the **smooth muscle** of the uterus. They are also called **uterine leiomyomas**. They are very common, affecting 40-60% of women in later reproductive years, and are more common in black women compared with other ethnic groups. They are **oestrogen sensitive**, meaning they grow in response to oestrogen.

Types

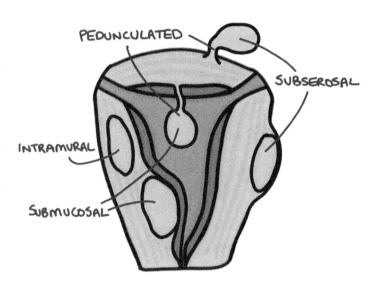

- *Intramural* means within the myometrium (the muscle of the uterus). As they grow, they change the shape and distort the uterus.
- *Subserosal* means just below the outer layer of the uterus. These fibroids grow outwards and can become very large, filling the abdominal cavity.
- *Submucosal* means just below the lining of the uterus (the endometrium).
- *Pedunculated* means on a stalk.

Presentation

Fibroids are often *asymptomatic*. They can present in several ways:
- **Heavy menstrual bleeding** (menorrhagia) is the most frequent presenting symptom
- Prolonged menstruation, lasting more than 7 days
- Abdominal pain, worse during menstruation
- Bloating or feeling full in the abdomen
- Urinary or bowel symptoms due to pelvic pressure or fullness
- Deep dyspareunia (pain during intercourse)
- Reduced fertility

Abdominal and **bimanual examination** may reveal a palpable pelvic mass or an enlarged firm non-tender uterus.

Investigations

- *Hysteroscopy* is the initial investigation for **submucosal fibroids** presenting with **heavy menstrual bleeding**.
- *Pelvic ultrasound* is the investigation of choice for larger fibroids.
- *MRI scanning* may be considered before surgical options, where more information is needed about the size, shape and blood supply of the fibroids.

Management

NICE guidelines on fibroids are included within the **heavy menstrual bleeding** guideline from 2018.

For fibroids **less than 3 cm**, the medical management is the same as with heavy menstrual bleeding:
- *Mirena coil* (first line) - fibroids must be less than 3cm with no distortion of the uterus
- *Symptomatic management* with NSAIDs and tranexamic acid
- *Combined oral contraceptive*
- *Cyclical oral progestogens*

Surgical options for managing smaller fibroids with heavy menstrual bleeding are:
- **Endometrial ablation**
- **Resection** of submucosal fibroids during hysteroscopy
- **Hysterectomy**

For fibroids **more than 3 cm**, women need **referral to gynaecology** for investigation and management. Medical options are:
- **Symptomatic** management with NSAIDs and tranexamic acid
- **Mirena coil** - depending on the size and shape of the fibroids and uterus
- **Combined oral contraceptive**
- **Cyclical oral progestogens**

Surgical options for larger fibroids are:
- **Uterine artery embolisation**
- **Myomectomy**
- **Hysterectomy**

GnRH agonists, such as **goserelin** (**Zoladex**) or **leuprorelin** (**Prostap**), may be used to reduce the size of fibroids before surgery. They work by inducing a menopause-like state and reducing the amount of oestrogen maintaining the fibroid. Usually, GnRH agonists are only used short term, for example, to shrink a fibroid before myomectomy.

Uterine Artery Embolisation

Uterine artery embolisation is a surgical option for larger fibroids, performed by *interventional radiologists*. The radiologist inserts a catheter into an artery, usually the **femoral artery**. This catheter is passed through to the **uterine artery** under X-ray guidance. Once in the correct place, particles are injected that cause a blockage in the arterial supply to the fibroid. This starves the fibroid of oxygen and causes it to shrink.

Surgical Options

Myomectomy involves surgically removing the fibroid via **laparoscopic** (keyhole) **surgery** or **laparotomy** (open surgery). Myomectomy is the only treatment known to potentially improve fertility in patients with fibroids.

Endometrial ablation can be used to destroy the endometrium. **Second generation**, non-hysteroscopic techniques are used, such as **balloon thermal ablation**. This involves inserting a specially designed balloon into the endometrial cavity and filling it with high-temperature fluid that burns the endometrial lining of the uterus.

Hysterectomy involves removing the uterus and fibroids. Hysterectomy may be by laparoscopy (keyhole surgery), laparotomy or vaginal approach. The ovaries may be removed or left depending on patient preference, risks and benefits.

Complications

There are several potential complications of fibroids:
- Heavy menstrual bleeding, often with iron deficiency anaemia
- Reduced fertility
- Pregnancy complications, such as miscarriages, premature labour and obstructive delivery
- Constipation
- Urinary outflow obstruction and urinary tract infections
- **Red degeneration** of the fibroid
- **Torsion** of the fibroid, usually affecting pedunculated fibroids
- **Malignant change** to a **leiomyosarcoma** is very rare (<1%)

Red Degeneration of Fibroids

Red degeneration refers to **ischaemia**, **infarction** and **necrosis** of the fibroid due to disrupted blood supply. Red degeneration is more likely to occur in larger fibroids (**above 5 cm**) during the second and third trimester of pregnancy. Red degeneration may occur as the fibroid rapidly enlarges during pregnancy, outgrowing its blood supply and becoming ischaemic. It may also occur due to kinking in the blood vessels as the uterus changes shape and expands during pregnancy.

Red degeneration presents with severe abdominal pain, low-grade fever, tachycardia and often vomiting. Management is supportive, with rest, fluids and analgesia.

TOM TIP: Look out for the pregnant woman with a history of fibroids presenting with severe abdominal pain and a low-grade fever in your exams. The diagnosis is likely to be red degeneration.

Endometriosis

Endometriosis is a condition where there is **ectopic endometrial tissue** outside the **uterus**. A lump of **endometrial tissue** outside the uterus is described as an **endometrioma**. **Endometriomas** in the **ovaries** are often called "**chocolate cysts**". **Adenomyosis** refers to endometrial tissue within the **myometrium** (muscle layer) of the uterus.

Aetiology

The exact cause of endometriosis is not clear, but there are several theories. No specific genes have been found to cause endometriosis; however, there does seem to be a genetic component to developing the condition.

One notable theory for the cause of ectopic endometrial tissue is that during menstruation, the endometrial lining flows backwards, through the **fallopian tubes** and out into the pelvis and peritoneum. This is called **retrograde menstruation**. The endometrial tissue then seeds itself around the pelvis and peritoneal cavity.

Other possible methods for endometrial tissue exiting the uterus have been proposed:
- **Embryonic cells** destined to become endometrial tissue may remain in areas outside the uterus during the development of the fetus, and later develop into ectopic endometrial tissue.
- There may be spread of endometrial cells through the **lymphatic system**, in a similar way to the spread of cancer.
- Cells outside the uterus somehow change, in a process called **metaplasia**, from typical cells of that organ into endometrial cells.

Pathophysiology of the Symptoms

The main symptom of endometriosis is **pelvic pain**. The cells of the endometrial tissue outside the uterus respond to hormones in the same way as endometrial tissue in the uterus. During menstruation, as the endometrial tissue in the uterus sheds its lining and bleeds, the same thing happens in the endometrial tissue elsewhere in the body. This causes irritation and inflammation of the tissues around the sites of endometriosis. This results in the cyclical, dull, heavy or burning pain that occurs during menstruation in patients with endometriosis.

Deposits of endometriosis in the bladder or bowel can lead to blood in the urine or stools.

Localised bleeding and inflammation can lead to **adhesions**. Inflammation causes damage and development of scar tissue that binds the organs together. For example, the ovaries may be fixed to the peritoneum, or the uterus may be fixed to the bowel. Adhesions can also occur after abdominal surgery. Adhesions lead to a **chronic**, **non-cyclical pain** that can be sharp, stabbing or pulling, and associated with nausea.

Endometriosis can lead to **reduced fertility**. Often it is not clear why women with endometriosis struggle to get pregnant. It may be due to adhesions around the ovaries and fallopian tubes, blocking the release of eggs or kinking the fallopian tubes and obstructing the route to the uterus. Endometriomas in the ovaries may also damage eggs or prevent effective ovulation.

Presentation

Endometriosis can be asymptomatic in some cases, or present with a number of symptoms:
- Cyclical abdominal or pelvic pain
- Deep dyspareunia (pain on deep sexual intercourse)
- Dysmenorrhoea (painful periods)
- Infertility
- Cyclical bleeding from other sites, such as haematuria

There can also be cyclical symptoms relating to other areas affected by the endometriosis:
- Urinary symptoms
- Bowel symptoms

Examination may reveal:
- Endometrial tissue visible in the vagina on speculum examination, particularly in the posterior fornix
- A fixed cervix on bimanual examination
- Tenderness in the vagina, cervix and adnexa

Diagnosis

Pelvic ultrasound may reveal large endometriomas and chocolate cysts. Ultrasound scans are often unremarkable in patients with endometriosis. Patients with suspected endometriosis need referral to a gynaecologist for laparoscopy.

Laparoscopic surgery is the **gold standard** way to diagnose abdominal and pelvic endometriosis. A definitive diagnosis can be established with a **biopsy** of the lesions during laparoscopy. Laparoscopy has the added benefit of allowing the surgeon to remove deposits of endometriosis and potentially improve symptoms.

Staging

The **American Society of Reproductive Medicine** (**ASRM**) has a staging system for endometriosis. It is worth being aware of this staging system; however, it is not mentioned in the **NICE guidelines**, and does not necessarily predict the symptoms or the difficulty in managing the condition. **NICE** recommend documenting a detailed description of the endometriosis rather than using a specific staging system. The ASRM staging system grades from least to most severe:
- Stage 1: Small superficial lesions
- Stage 2: Mild, but deeper lesions than stage 1
- Stage 3: Deeper lesions, with lesions on the ovaries and mild adhesions
- Stage 4: Deep and large lesions affecting the ovaries with extensive adhesions

Management

Helpful guidelines for the management of endometriosis are the *RCOG Green-top guideline 41* on *chronic pelvic pain* (2012), the *ESHRE guidelines* on *endometriosis* (2013) and the *NICE clinical knowledge summaries* (2020).

Initial management involves:
- Establishing a diagnosis
- Providing a clear explanation
- Listening to the patient, establishing their ideas, concerns and expectations and building a partnership
- Analgesia as required for pain (NSAIDs and paracetamol first line)

Hormonal management options can be tried before establishing a definitive diagnosis with laparoscopy:
- Combined oral contractive pill, which can be used back-to-back without a pill-free period if helpful
- Progestogen-only pill
- Medroxyprogesterone acetate injection (e.g. Depo-Provera)
- Nexplanon implant
- Mirena coil
- GnRH agonists

Surgical management options:
- Laparoscopic surgery to *excise* or *ablate* the endometrial tissue and remove adhesions (*adhesiolysis*)
- Hysterectomy

Laparoscopic treatment may improve fertility. Hormonal therapies may improve symptoms but not fertility.

Explanation of Treatment Options

Cyclical pain can be treated with hormonal medications that *stop ovulation* and *reduce endometrial thickening*. This can be achieved using the combined oral contraceptive pill, oral progestogen-only pill, the progestogen depot injection, the progestogen implant (Nexplanon) or the Mirena coil.

The cyclical pain tends to improve after the menopause when the female sex hormones are reduced. Therefore, another treatment option for endometriosis is to induce a *menopause-like state* using *GnRH agonists*. Examples of GnRH agonists are *goserelin* (*Zoladex*) or *leuprorelin* (*Prostap*). They shut down the ovaries temporarily and can be useful in treating pain in many women. However, inducing the menopause has several side effects, such as hot flushes, night sweats and a risk of *osteoporosis*.

Laparoscopic surgery can be used to *excise* or *ablate* the ectopic endometrial tissue. In women where there is chronic pelvic pain due to *adhesions*, surgery can be used to dissect the adhesions and attempt to return the anatomy to normal.

Hysterectomy and bilateral salpingo-opherectomy is the final surgical option. During the procedure, the surgeon will attempt to remove as much of the endometriosis as possible. Importantly, this is still not guaranteed to resolve symptoms. Removing the ovaries induces menopause, and this stops ectopic endometrial tissue responding to the menstrual cycle.

Infertility secondary to endometriosis can be treated with surgery. The aim is to remove as much of the endometriosis as possible, treat adhesions and return the anatomy to normal. This improves fertility in some but not all women with endometriosis.

Adenomyosis

Adenomyosis refers to **endometrial tissue** inside the **myometrium** (muscle layer of the uterus). It is more common in later reproductive years and those that have had several pregnancies (**multiparous**). It occurs in around 10% of women overall. It may occur alone, or alongside endometriosis or fibroids. The cause is not fully understood, and multiple factors are involved, including sex hormones, trauma and inflammation. The condition is hormone-dependent, and symptoms tend to resolve after menopause, similarly to endometriosis and fibroids.

Presentation

Adenomyosis typically presents with:
- Painful periods (**dysmenorrhoea**)
- Heavy periods (**menorrhagia**)
- Pain during intercourse (**dyspareunia**)

It may also present with infertility or pregnancy-related complications. Around a third of patients are asymptomatic.

Examination can demonstrate an enlarged and tender uterus. It will feel more soft than a uterus containing fibroids.

Diagnosis

Transvaginal ultrasound of the pelvis is the first-line investigation for suspected adenomyosis.

MRI and **transabdominal ultrasound** are alternative investigations where transvaginal ultrasound is not suitable.

The gold standard is to perform a **histological examination** of the uterus after a hysterectomy. However, this is not usually a suitable way of establishing the diagnosis for obvious reasons.

Management

Management of adenomyosis will depend on symptoms, age and plans for pregnancy. NICE recommend the same treatment for adenomyosis as for heavy menstrual bleeding.

When the woman does **not** want contraception; treatment can be used during menstruation for symptomatic relief, with:
- Tranexamic acid when there is no associated pain (antifibrinolytic - reduces bleeding)
- Mefenamic acid when there is associated pain (NSAID - reduces bleeding and pain)

Management when contraception is wanted or acceptable:
1. Mirena coil (first line)
2. Combined oral contraceptive pill
3. Cyclical oral progestogens

Progesterone only medications such as the pill, implant or depot injection may also be helpful.

Other options are that may be considered by a specialist include:
- GnRH analogues to induce a menopause-like state
- Endometrial ablation
- Uterine artery embolisation
- Hysterectomy

Pregnancy and Adenomyosis

Adenomyosis is associated with:
- Infertility
- Miscarriage
- Preterm birth
- Small for gestational age
- Preterm premature rupture of membranes
- Malpresentation
- Need for caesarean section
- Postpartum haemorrhage

Menopause

Menopause is a **retrospective diagnosis**, made after a woman has had no periods for **12 months**. It is defined as a permanent end to menstruation. On average, women experience the menopause around the age of 51 years, although this can vary significantly. Menopause is a normal process affecting all women reaching a suitable age.

Menopause is the point at which menstruation stops.

Postmenopause describes the period from 12 months after the final menstrual period onwards.

Perimenopause refers to the time around the menopause, where the woman may be experiencing **vasomotor symptoms** and **irregular periods**. *Perimenopause* includes the time leading up to the last menstrual period, and the 12 months afterwards. This is typically in women older than 45 years.

Premature menopause is menopause before the age of 40 years. It is the result of **premature ovarian insufficiency**.

Menopause is caused by a lack of **ovarian follicular function**, resulting in changes in the sex hormones associated with the menstrual cycle:
- **Oestrogen** and **progesterone** levels are **low**
- **LH** and **FSH** levels are **high**, in response to an **absence** of negative feedback from oestrogen

Physiology

Inside the ovaries, the process of **primordial follicles** maturing into **primary** and **secondary follicles** is always occurring, independent of the menstrual cycle. At the start of the menstrual cycle, **FSH** stimulates further development of the **secondary follicles**. As the follicles grow, the **granulosa cells** that surround them secrete increasing amounts of **oestrogen**.

The process of menopause begins with a decline in the development of the ovarian **follicles**. Without the growth of follicles, there is reduced production of **oestrogen**. Oestrogen has a **negative feedback** effect on the **pituitary gland**, suppressing the quantity of **LH** and **FSH** produced. As the level of oestrogen falls in the perimenopausal period, there is an **absence** of **negative feedback** on the **pituitary gland**, and increasing levels of **LH** and **FSH**.

The failing follicular development means ovulation does not occur (**anovulation**), resulting in irregular menstrual cycles. Without oestrogen, the endometrium does not develop, leading to a lack of menstruation (**amenorrhoea**). Lower levels of oestrogen also cause the **perimenopausal symptoms**.

Perimenopausal Symptoms

A lack of oestrogen in the perimenopausal period leads to symptoms of:
- Hot flushes
- Emotional lability or low mood
- Premenstrual syndrome
- Irregular periods
- Joint pains
- Heavier or lighter periods
- Vaginal dryness and atrophy
- Reduced libido

Risks

A lack of oestrogen increases the risk of certain conditions:
- Cardiovascular disease and stroke
- Osteoporosis
- Pelvic organ prolapse
- Urinary incontinence

Diagnosis

A diagnosis of **perimenopause** and **menopause** can be made in women **over 45 years** with typical symptoms, without performing any investigations.

NICE guidelines (2015) recommend considering an **FSH blood test** to help with the diagnosis in:
- Women under 40 years with suspected premature menopause
- Women aged 40 - 45 years with menopausal symptoms or a change in the menstrual cycle

Contraception

Fertility gradually declines after 40 years of age. However, women should still consider themselves fertile. Pregnancy after 40 is associated with increased risks and complications. Women need to use effective contraception for:
- Two years after the last menstrual period in women under 50
- One year after the last menstrual period in women over 50

Hormonal contraceptives do not affect the menopause, when it occurs or how long it lasts, although they may suppress and mask the symptoms. This can make diagnosing menopause in women on hormonal contraception more difficult.

Good contraceptive options (**UKMEC 1**, meaning no restrictions) for women approaching the menopause are:
- Barrier methods
- Mirena or copper coil
- Progestogen-only pill
- Progestogen implant
- Progestogen depot injection (under 45 years)
- Sterilisation

The **combined oral contraceptive pill** is **UKMEC 2** (the advantages generally outweigh the risks) after aged 40, and can be used up to age 50 years if there are no other contraindications. Consider combined oral contraceptive pills containing **norethisterone** or **levonorgestrel** in women over 40, due to the relatively lower risk of **venous thromboembolism** compared with other options.

TOM TIP: It is worth making a note and remembering two key side effects of the progestogen depot injection (e.g. Depo-Provera): weight gain and reduced bone mineral density (osteoporosis). These side effects are unique to the depot and do not occur with other forms of contraception. Reduced bone mineral density makes the depot unsuitable for women over 45 years.

Management of Perimenopausal Symptoms

Vasomotor symptoms are likely to resolve after 2 - 5 years without any treatment. Management of symptoms depends on the severity, personal circumstances and response to treatment. Options include:
- No treatment
- **Hormone replacement therapy** (HRT)
- **Tibolone**, a synthetic steroid hormone that acts as continuous combined HRT (only after 12 months of amenorrhoea)
- **Clonidine**, which act as an agonist of alpha-adrenergic and imidazoline receptors
- **Cognitive behavioural therapy** (CBT)
- **SSRI antidepressants**, such as fluoxetine or citalopram
- **Testosterone** can be used to treat reduced libido (usually as a gel or cream)
- **Vaginal oestrogen** cream or tablets, to help with vaginal dryness and atrophy (can be used alongside systemic HRT)
- **Vaginal moisturisers**, such as Sylk, Replens and YES

Premature Ovarian Insufficiency

Premature ovarian insufficiency is defined as menopause before the age of 40 years. It is the result of a decline in the normal activity of the ovaries at an early age. It presents with early onset of the typical symptoms of the menopause.

Premature ovarian insufficiency is characterised by **hypergonadotropic hypogonadism**. Under-activity of the gonads (**hypogonadism**) means there is a **lack** of **negative feedback** on the **pituitary gland**, resulting in an excess of the gonadotropins (**hypergonadotropism**). Hormonal analysis will show:
- Raised LH and FSH levels (gonadotropins)
- Low oestradiol levels

Causes

- **Idiopathic** (the cause is unknown in more than 50% of cases)
- **Iatrogenic**, due to interventions such as chemotherapy, radiotherapy or surgery (i.e. oophorectomy)
- **Autoimmune**, possibly associated with coeliac disease, adrenal insufficiency, type 1 diabetes or thyroid disease
- **Genetic**, with a positive family history or conditions such as Turner's syndrome
- **Infections** such as mumps, tuberculosis or cytomegalovirus

Presentation

Premature ovarian insufficiency presents with **irregular menstrual periods**, lack of menstrual periods (**secondary amenorrhea**) and symptoms of **low oestrogen levels**, such has hot flushes, night sweats and vaginal dryness.

Diagnosis

NICE guidelines on menopause (2015) say premature ovarian insufficiency can be diagnosed in women **younger than 40 years** with **typical menopausal symptoms** plus **elevated FSH**.

The FSH level needs to be persistently raised (more than 25 IU/l) on two consecutive samples separated by more than four weeks to make a diagnosis. The results are difficult to interpret in women taking hormonal contraception.

Associations

Women with premature ovarian failure are at higher risk of multiple conditions relating to the lack of oestrogen, including:
- Cardiovascular disease
- Stroke
- Osteoporosis
- Cognitive impairment
- Dementia
- Parkinsonism

Management

Management involves **hormone replacement therapy** (**HRT**) until at least the age at which women typically go through menopause. HRT reduces the cardiovascular, osteoporosis, cognitive and psychological risks associated with premature menopause. It is worth noting there is still a small risk of pregnancy in women with premature ovarian failure, and contraception is still required.

There are two options for HRT in women with premature ovarian insufficiency:
- Traditional hormone replacement therapy
- Combined oral contraceptive pill

Traditional hormone replacement therapy is associated with a **lower blood pressure** compared with the combined oral contraceptive pill. The combined pill may be more socially acceptable (**less stigma** for younger women). It also acts as **contraception**.

Hormone replacement therapy before the age of 50 is not considered to increase the risk of **breast cancer** compared with the general population, as women would ordinarily produce the same hormones at this age.

There may be an increased risk of **venous thromboembolism** with HRT in women under 50 years. The risk of VTE can be reduced by using transdermal methods (i.e. patches).

Hormone Replacement Therapy

Hormone replacement therapy (**HRT**) is used in **perimenopausal** and **postmenopausal** women to alleviate symptoms associated with the menopause. These symptoms are associated with a declined in the level of oestrogen. **Exogenous oestrogen** is given to alleviate the symptoms.

Progesterone needs to be given (in addition to oestrogen) to women that **have a uterus**. The primary purpose of adding **progesterone** is to prevent **endometrial hyperplasia** and **endometrial cancer** secondary to "**unopposed**" oestrogen.

Not all menopausal women require hormone replacement therapy. Women have often tried non-hormonal methods of controlling their symptoms before seeking help from their GP. HRT can offer very effective relief from symptoms, and in the majority of women the benefits will outweigh the risks.

TOM TIP: Hormone replacement therapy is a massive topic. If you remember one thing about HRT for your exams, remember the basics of choosing the HRT regime. Women with a uterus require endometrial protection with progesterone, whereas women without a uterus can have oestrogen-only HRT. Women that still have periods should go on cyclical HRT, with cyclical progesterone and regular breakthrough bleeds. Postmenopausal women with a uterus and more than 12 months without periods should go on continuous combined HRT.

Non-Hormonal Treatments for Menopausal Symptoms

Non-hormonal treatments may be tried initially, or used when there are contraindications to HRT. Options include:
- **Lifestyle changes** such as improving the diet, exercise, weight loss, smoking cessation, reducing alcohol, reducing caffeine and reducing stress
- **Cognitive behavioural therapy** (CBT)
- **Clonidine**, which is an agonist of alpha-adrenergic and imidazoline receptors
- **SSRI antidepressants** (e.g. fluoxetine)
- **Venlafaxine**, which is a selective serotonin-norepinephrine reuptake inhibitor (SNRI)
- **Gabapentin**

Clonidine

Clonidine act as an **agonist** of **alpha-2 adrenergic receptors** and **imidazoline receptors** in the brain. It lowers blood pressure and reduces the heart rate, and is also used as an antihypertensive medication. It can be helpful for **vasomotor symptoms** and **hot flushes**, particularly where there are contraindications to using HRT.

Common side effects of clonidine are dry mouth, headaches, dizziness and fatigue. Sudden withdrawal can result in rapid increases in blood pressure and agitation.

Alternative Remedies

Patients might try alternative remedies, although they are not generally recommended as the safety and efficacy is unclear. They can have significant side effects and interact with other medications. These alternative remedies are intended to manage the vasomotor symptoms, such as hot flushes:
- **Black cohosh**, which may be a cause of liver damage
- **Dong quai**, which may cause bleeding disorders
- **Red clover**, which may have oestrogenic effects that would be concerning with oestrogen sensitive cancers
- **Evening primrose oil**, which has significant drug interactions and is linked with clotting disorders and seizures
- **Ginseng** may be used for mood and sleep benefits

Indications for HRT

The indications for HRT are:
- Replacing hormones in **premature ovarian insufficiency**, even without symptoms
- Reducing **vasomotor symptoms** such as hot flushes and night sweats
- Improving symptoms such as **low mood**, **decreased libido**, **poor sleep** and **joint pain**
- Reducing the risk of **osteoporosis** in women under 60 years

Benefits of HRT

In women under 60 years, the benefits of HRT generally outweigh the risks.

The key benefits to inform women of include:
- Improved vasomotor and other symptoms of the menopause (including mood, urogenital and joint symptoms)
- Improved quality of life
- Reduced risk of osteoporosis and fractures

Risks of HRT

Women may be concerned about the risks of HRT. It is crucial to put these into perspective. In women under 60 years, the benefits generally outweigh the risks. Specific treatment regimes significantly reduce the risks associated with HRT.

The risks of HRT are more significant in older women, and increase with longer duration of treatment. The principal risks of HRT are:
- Increased risk of **breast cancer**
- Increased risk of **endometrial cancer**
- Increased risk of **venous thromboembolism** (2 - 3 times the background risk)
- Increased risk of **stroke** and **coronary artery disease** with long-term use in older women
- The evidence is inconclusive about **ovarian cancer**, and if there is an increase in risk, it is minimal

These risks do not apply to all women:
- The risks are not increased in **women under 50 years** compared with other women their age
- There is no risk of **endometrial cancer** in women **without a uterus**
- There is no increased risk of **breast cancer** with **oestrogen-only HRT** (the risk may even be reduced on treatment)
- There is no increased risk of **cardiovascular disease** with **oestrogen-only HRT** (the risk may even be lower with HRT)

Ways to reduce the risks:
- The risk of **endometrial cancer** is greatly reduced by **adding progestogens** in women with a uterus
- The risk of **VTE** is reduced by using **patches** rather than pills
- The risk of **breast cancer** can be reduced by using **local progestogens** (i.e. Mirena coil) rather than systemic
- The risk of **cardiovascular disease** can be reduced by using **local progestogens** (i.e. Mirena coil) rather than systemic

Contraindications to HRT

There are some essential contraindications to consider in patients wanting to start HRT:
- Undiagnosed abnormal bleeding
- Endometrial hyperplasia or cancer
- Breast cancer
- Uncontrolled hypertension
- Venous thromboembolism
- Liver disease
- Active angina or myocardial infarction
- Pregnancy

Assessment Before HRT

Before initiating HRT, there are a few things to check and consider:
- Take a full history to ensure there are no contraindications
- Take a family history to assess the risk of **oestrogen dependent cancers** (e.g. breast cancer) and **VTE**
- Check the body mass index (BMI) and blood pressure
- Ensure cervical and breast screening is up to date
- Encourage lifestyle changes that are likely to improve symptoms and reduce risks

Choosing the HRT Formulation

There are three steps to consider when choosing the HRT formulation:

Step 1: Do they have local or systemic symptoms?
- Local symptoms: use **topical treatments** such as topical oestrogen cream or tablets
- Systemic symptoms: use **systemic treatment** - go to step 2

Step 2: Does the woman have a uterus?
- No uterus: use continuous **oestrogen-only** HRT
- Has uterus: add **progesterone** (**combined** HRT) - go to step 3

Step 3: Have they had a period in the past 12 months?
- **Perimenopausal**: give **cyclical combined HRT**
- **Postmenopausal** (more than 12 months since last period): give **continuous combined HRT**

Options for Oestrogen Delivery

Oestrogen is the critical component of HRT for reducing the symptoms of menopause. There are two options for delivering systemic oestrogen:
- Oral (tablets)
- Transdermal (patches or gels)

Patches are more suitable for women with poor control on oral treatment, higher risk of venous thromboembolism, cardiovascular disease and headaches.

Options for Progesterone Delivery

Progesterone is added to HRT to reduce the risk of **endometrial hyperplasia** and **endometrial cancer**. Progesterone is only required in women that have a uterus. Women **without** a uterus do not need progesterone, and can have **oestrogen-only HRT**.

Cyclical progesterone, given for 10 - 14 days per month, is used for women that have had a period within the past 12 months. Cycling the progesterone allows patients to have a monthly breakthrough bleed during the oestrogen-only part of the cycle, similar to a period.

Continuous progesterone is used when the woman has not had a period in the past:
- 24 months if under 50 years
- 12 months if over 50 years

Using **continuous combined HRT** before postmenopause can lead to irregular breakthrough bleeding, leading to investigations for other underlying causes of bleeding.

You can switch from **cyclical** to **continuous** HRT after at least 12 months of treatment in women over 50, and 24 months in women under 50. Switch from cyclical to continuous HRT during the withdrawal bleed. Continuous HRT has better endometrial protection than cyclical HRT.

There are three options for delivering progesterone for endometrial protection:
- **Oral** (tablets)
- **Transdermal** (patches)
- **Intrauterine system** (e.g. Mirena coil)

Cyclical combined HRT options include **sequential** tablets or patches containing continuous oestrogen, with progesterone added for specific periods during the cycle.

The **Mirena coil** is licensed for four years for **endometrial protection**, after which time it needs replacing. The Mirena coil has the added benefits of **contraception** and treating **heavy menstrual periods**. It can cause irregular bleeding and spotting in the first few months after insertion. This usually settles with time and many women become amenorrhoeic.

Types of Progesterone

The terms around progesterone can be confusing. There are some key definitions to remember:
- **Progestogens** refer to any chemicals that target and stimulate progesterone receptors
- **Progesterone** is the hormone produced naturally in the body
- **Progestins** are synthetic progestogens

There are two significant **progestogen classes** used in HRT. If the woman experiences side effects, consider switching the progestogen class. They can be described as **C19** and **C21 progestogens**, referring to the chemical structure and number of carbon atoms in the molecule.

C19 progestogens are derived from **testosterone**, and are more "male" in their effects. Examples are **norethisterone**, **levonorgestrel** and **desogestrel**. These may be helpful for women with **reduced libido**.

C21 progestogens are derived from **progesterone**, and are more "female" in their effects. Examples are **progesterone**, **dydrogesterone** and **medroxyprogesterone**. These may be helpful for women with side effects such as depressed mood or acne.

Example Regimes

In a women with no uterus:
- Oestrogen-only pills, for example, **Elleste Solo** or **Premarin**
- Oestrogen-only patches, for example, **Evorel** or **Estradot**

In a perimenopausal woman with periods:
- Cyclical combined **tablets**, for example, **Elleste-Duet**, **Clinorette** or **Femoston**
- Cyclical combined **patches**, for example, **Evorel Sequi** or **FemSeven Sequi**
- **Mirena coil** plus oestrogen-only pills, for example, **Elleste Solo** or **Premarin**
- **Mirena coil** plus oestrogen-only patches, for example, **Evorel** or **Estradot**

In a postmenopausal woman with a uterus:
- Continuous combined **tablets**, for example, **Elleste-Duet Conti**, **Kliofem** or **Femoston Conti**
- Continuous combined **patches**, for example, **Evorel-Conti** or **FemSeven Conti**
- **Mirena coil** plus oestrogen-only pills, for example, **Elleste Solo** or **Premarin**
- **Mirena coil** plus oestrogen-only patches, for example, **Evorel** or **Estradot**

TOM TIP: The key to HRT is to remember the principles, so that you can counsel women and look up the specific regimes when required. The best way of delivering oestrogen is with patches, due to the reduced risk of venous-thromboembolism. The best way of providing progesterone is with an intrauterine device, for example, the Mirena coil. The coil has the added benefits of contraception and treating heavy menstrual periods. Additionally, women will not experience progestogenic side effects, or the increased risk of breast cancer and cardiovascular disease associated with systemic progesterone with combined HRT.

Tibolone

Tibolone is a **synthetic steroid** that stimulates **oestrogen** and **progesterone receptors**. It also weakly stimulates **androgen receptors**. The effects on androgen receptors mean tibolone can be helpful for patients with **reduced libido**.

Tibolone is used as a form of **continuous combined HRT**. Women need to be more than 12 months without a period (24 months if under 50 years). They would be expected not to have breakthrough bleeding. Tibolone can cause irregular bleeding, resulting in further investigations to exclude other causes.

Testosterone

Testosterone is a male sex hormone (**androgen**). It is naturally present in low levels in women. Menopause can be associated with reduced testosterone, resulting in low energy and reduced libido (sex drive). Treatment with testosterone is usually initiated and monitored by a specialist. It is given by **transdermal** application, applied as a gel or a cream to the skin.

Additional Management Points

- Follow-up three months after initiating HRT to review symptom and side effects
- Side effects often settle with time, so it is worth persisting for at least three months with each regime
- It takes 3 - 6 months of treatment to gain the full effects
- Problematic or irregular bleeding is an indication for referral to a specialist
- Ensure the woman has appropriate contraception
- Stop oestrogen-containing contraceptives or HRT **4 weeks before major surgery** (NICE guidelines 2018 - NG89)
- Consider other causes of symptoms where they persist despite HRT (e.g. thyroid, liver disease and diabetes)

Contraception with HRT

Hormone replacement therapy does not act as contraception. It is important to ensure perimenopausal women have adequate contraception. Common options are:
- **Mirena coil**
- **Progestogen-only pill**, given in addition to HRT

Side effects

The oestrogen and progesterone components of HRT cause different side effects.

Oestrogenic side effects:
- Nausea and bloating
- Breast swelling
- Breast tenderness
- Headaches
- Leg cramps

Progestogenic side effects:
- Mood swings
- Bloating
- Fluid retention
- Weight gain
- Acne and greasy skin

Where patients experience side effects, it is worth changing the type of HRT or the route of administration (switch between patches and pills).

Patients with progestogenic side effects may do better switching to a HRT with a different form of progesterone. For example, patients with acne and mood swings may do better with a **dydrogesterone** progesterone (e.g. **Femoston**). In contrast, patients with reduced libido may do better with a **norethisterone** progesterone (e.g. **Elleste-Duet**). Progestogenic side effects can be avoided altogether by using a Mirena coil for endometrial protection.

Unscheduled bleeding can occur in the first 3 - 6 months of HRT (in women with a uterus). If unscheduled bleeding continues, consider referral for investigations, particularly regarding endometrial cancer.

Stopping HRT

There is no specific regime for stopping HRT. It can be reduced gradually or stopped abruptly, depending on the preference of the woman. This choice does not affect long term symptoms. Gradually reducing the HRT may be preferable to reduce the risk of symptoms recurring suddenly.

Polycystic Ovarian Syndrome

Polycystic ovarian syndrome (**PCOS**) is a common condition causing metabolic and reproductive problems in women. There are characteristic features of **multiple ovarian cysts**, **infertility**, **oligomenorrhea**, **hyperandrogenism** and **insulin resistance**.

There are some essential definitions to be aware of with polycystic ovarian syndrome:
- **Anovulation** refers to the absence of ovulation
- **Oligoovulation** refers to irregular, infrequent ovulation
- **Amenorrhoea** refers to the absence of menstrual periods
- **Oligomenorrhoea** refers to irregular, infrequent menstrual periods
- **Androgens** are male sex hormones, such as testosterone
- **Hyperandrogenism** refers to the effects of high levels of androgens
- **Hirsutism** refers to the growth of thick dark hair, often in a male pattern, for example, male pattern facial hair
- **Insulin resistance** refers to a lack of response to the hormone insulin, resulting in high blood sugar levels

Rotterdam Criteria

The Rotterdam criteria are used for making a diagnosis of polycystic ovarian syndrome. A diagnosis requires at least two of the three key features:
- **Oligoovulation** or **anovulation**, presenting with irregular or absent menstrual periods
- **Hyperandrogenism**, characterised by hirsutism and acne
- **Polycystic ovaries** on **ultrasound** (or ovarian volume of more than 10cm^3)

TOM TIP: If you are going to remember one thing about polycystic ovarian syndrome, remember the triad of anovulation, hyperandrogenism and polycystic ovaries on ultrasound. The Rotterdam criteria are commonly tested in MCQs and asked by examiners in OSCEs. It is important to remember that only having one of these three features does not meet the criteria for a diagnosis. As many as 20% of reproductive age women have multiple small cysts on their ovaries. Unless they also have anovulation or hyperandrogenism, they do not have polycystic ovarian syndrome.

Presentation

Women with polycystic ovarian syndrome present with some key features:
- Oligomenorrhoea or amenorrhoea
- Infertility
- Obesity (in about 70% of patients with PCOS)
- Hirsutism
- Acne
- Hair loss in a male pattern

Other Features and Complications

In addition to the presenting features, women may also experience:
- Insulin resistance and diabetes
- Acanthosis nigricans
- Cardiovascular disease
- Hypercholesterolaemia
- Endometrial hyperplasia and cancer
- Obstructive sleep apnoea
- Depression and anxiety
- Sexual problems

Acanthosis nigricans describes thickened, rough skin, typically found in the axilla and on the elbows. It has a velvety texture. It occurs with **insulin resistance**.

Differential Diagnosis of Hirsutism

An important feature of polycystic ovarian syndrome is **hirsutism**. Hirsutism can also be caused by:
- **Medications**, such as phenytoin, ciclosporin, corticosteroids, testosterone and anabolic steroids
- **Ovarian** or **adrenal tumours** that secrete androgens
- **Cushing's syndrome**
- **Congenital adrenal hyperplasia**

Insulin Resistance

Insulin resistance is a crucial part of PCOS. When someone is resistant to insulin, their **pancreas** has to produce **more insulin** to get a response from the cells of the body. Insulin promotes the release of **androgens** from the **ovaries** and **adrenal glands**. Therefore, higher levels of insulin result in higher levels of **androgens** (such as **testosterone**). Insulin also suppresses **sex hormone-binding globulin** (**SHBG**) production by the **liver**. SHBG normally binds to androgens and suppresses their function. Reduced SHBG further promotes **hyperandrogenism** in women with PCOS.

The high insulin levels contribute to halting the development of the **follicles** in the **ovaries**, leading to anovulation and multiple partially developed follicles (seen as polycystic ovaries on the scan).

Diet, **exercise** and **weight** loss help reduce insulin resistance.

Investigations

The **NICE clinical knowledge summaries** recommend the following **blood tests** to diagnose PCOS and exclude other pathology that may have a similar presentation:
- Testosterone
- Sex hormone-binding globulin
- Luteinizing hormone
- Follicle-stimulating hormone
- Prolactin (may be mildly elevated in PCOS)
- Thyroid-stimulating hormone

Hormonal blood tests typically show:
- **Raised luteinising hormone**
- **Raised LH to FSH ratio** (high LH compared with FSH)
- **Raised testosterone**
- Raised insulin
- Normal or raised oestrogen levels

TOM TIP: The key thing to remember for your exams is the raised LH, and the raised LH:FSH ratio.

Pelvic ultrasound is required when suspecting PCOS. A **transvaginal ultrasound** is the gold standard for visualising the ovaries. The **follicles** may be arranged around the periphery of the ovary, giving a **"string of pearls"** appearance. The diagnostic criteria are either:
- 12 or more developing follicles in one ovary
- Ovarian volume of more than 10cm^3

Pelvic ultrasound is not reliable in **adolescents** for the diagnosis of PCOS.

TOM TIP: It is worth remembering the "string of pearls" description for your exams. It may come up in MCQs. It is also worth remembering that an ovarian volume of more than 10cm^3 can indicate polycystic ovarian syndrome, even without the presence of cysts.

The screening test of choice for diabetes in patients with PCOS is a 2-hour 75g **oral glucose tolerance test** (**OGTT**). An OGTT is performed in the morning prior to having breakfast. It involves taking a baseline **fasting plasma glucose**, giving a **75g glucose drink** and then measuring plasma glucose **2 hours later**. It tests the ability of the body to cope with a carbohydrate meal. The results are:
- **Impaired fasting glucose** - fasting glucose of 6.1 – 6.9 mmol/l (before the glucose drink)
- **Impaired glucose tolerance** - plasma glucose at 2 hours of 7.8 – 11.1 mmol/l
- **Diabetes** - plasma glucose at 2 hours above 11.1 mmol/l

General Management

It is crucial to reduce the risks associated with **obesity**, **type 2 diabetes**, **hypercholesterolaemia** and **cardiovascular disease**. These risks can be reduced by:
- Weight loss
- Low glycaemic index, calorie-controlled diet
- Exercise
- Smoking cessation
- Antihypertensive medications where required
- Statins where indicated (QRISK >10%)

Patients should be assessed and managed for the associated features and complications, such as:
- Endometrial hyperplasia and cancer
- Infertility
- Hirsutism
- Acne
- Obstructive sleep apnoea
- Depression and anxiety

Weight loss is a significant part of the management of PCOS. Weight loss alone can result in ovulation and restore fertility and regular menstruation, improve insulin resistance, reduce hirsutism and reduce the risks of associated conditions. **Orlistat** may be used to help weight loss in women with a BMI above 30. Orlistat is a **lipase inhibitor** that stops the absorption of fat in the intestines.

Managing the Risk of Endometrial Cancer

Women with polycystic ovarian syndrome have several risk factors for **endometrial cancer**:
- Obesity
- Diabetes
- Insulin resistance
- Amenorrhoea

Under normal circumstances, the **corpus luteum** releases **progesterone** after ovulation. Women with PCOS do not ovulate (or ovulate infrequently), and therefore do not produce sufficient progesterone. They continue to produce oestrogen and do not experience regular menstruation. Consequently, the endometrial lining continues to proliferate under the influence of oestrogen, without regular shedding during menstruation. This is similar to giving **unopposed** *oestrogen* in women on hormone replacement therapy. It results in **endometrial hyperplasia** and a significant risk of **endometrial cancer**.

Women with **extended gaps** between periods (more than three months) or **abnormal bleeding** need to be investigated with a **pelvic ultrasound** to assess the **endometrial thickness**. **Cyclical progestogens** should be used to induce a period **prior to** the ultrasound scan. If the endometrial thickness is more than 10mm, they need to be referred for a biopsy to exclude endometrial hyperplasia or cancer.

Options for reducing the risk of endometrial hyperplasia and endometrial cancer are:
- *Mirena coil* for continuous endometrial protection
- *Inducing a withdrawal bleed* at least every 3 - 4 months with either:
  - *Cyclical progestogens* (e.g. medroxyprogesterone acetate 10mg once a day for 14 days)
  - *Combined oral contraceptive pill*

Managing Infertility

Weight loss is the initial step for improving fertility. Losing weight can restore regular ovulation.

A specialist may initiate other options where weight loss fails. These include:
- Clomifene
- Laparoscopic ovarian drilling
- In vitro fertilisation (IVF)

Metformin and *letrozole* may also help restore ovulation under the guidance of a specialist; however, the evidence to support their use is not clear.

Ovarian drilling involves **laparoscopic surgery**. The surgeon punctures multiple holes in the ovaries using **diathermy** or **laser therapy**. This can improve the woman's hormonal profile and result in regular ovulation and fertility.

Women that become pregnant require screening for **gestational diabetes**. Screening involves an **oral glucose tolerance test**, performed before pregnancy and at 24 - 28 weeks gestation.

Managing Hirsutism

Weight loss may improve the symptoms of hirsutism. Women are likely to have already explored options for hair removal, such as waxing, shaving and plucking.

Co-cyprindiol (**Dianette**) is a **combined oral contraceptive pill** licensed for the treatment of **hirsutism** and **acne**. It has an **anti-androgenic effect**, works as a contraceptive and will also regulate periods. The downside is a significantly increased risk of **venous thromboembolism**. For this reason, co-cyprindiol is usually stopped after three months of use.

Topical eflornithine can be used to treat facial hirsutism. It usually takes 6 - 8 weeks to see a significant improvement. The hirsutism will return within two months of stopping eflornithine.

Other options that may be considered by a specialist experienced in treating hirsutism include:
- *Electrolysis*
- *Laser hair removal*
- *Spironolactone* (mineralocorticoid antagonist with anti-androgen effects)
- *Finasteride* (5α-reductase inhibitor that decreases testosterone production)
- *Flutamide* (non-steroidal anti-androgen)
- *Cyproterone acetate* (anti-androgen and progestin)

Management of Acne

The **combined oral contraceptive pill** is first-line for acne in PCOS. Co-cyprindiol may be the best option as it has anti-androgen effects; however, there is a significantly increased risk of **venous thromboembolism**.

Other standard treatments for acne include:
- Topical **adapalene** (a retinoid)
- Topical **antibiotics** (e.g. clindamycin 1% with benzoyl peroxide 5%)
- Topical **azelaic acid 20%**
- Oral **tetracycline antibiotics** (e.g. lymecycline)

Ovarian Cysts

A cyst is a **fluid-filled sac**. **Functional ovarian cysts** relate to the fluctuating hormones of the menstrual cycle, and are very common in **premenopausal** women. The vast majority of ovarian cysts in **premenopausal** women are benign. Cysts in **postmenopausal** women are more concerning for **malignancy** and need further investigation.

Patients with **multiple ovarian cysts** or a "**string of pearls**" appearance to the ovaries cannot be diagnosed with **polycystic ovarian syndrome** unless they also have other features of the condition. A diagnosis of PCOS requires at least two of:
- Anovulation
- Hyperandrogenism
- Polycystic ovaries on ultrasound

Presentation

Most ovarian cysts are asymptomatic. Cysts are often found incidentally on pelvic ultrasound scans.

Occasionally, ovarian cysts can cause non-specific symptoms of:
- Pelvic pain
- Bloating
- Fullness in the abdomen
- A palpable pelvic mass (particularly with very large cysts such as mucinous cystadenomas)

Ovarian cysts may present with acute pelvic pain if there is **ovarian torsion**, **haemorrhage** or **rupture** of the cyst.

Functional Cysts

Follicular cysts represent the developing follicle. When these fail to rupture and release the egg, the cyst can persist. Follicular cysts are the most common ovarian cyst, they are harmless and tend to disappear after a few menstrual cycles. Typically they have thin walls and no internal structures, giving a reassuring appearance on the ultrasound.

Corpus luteum cysts occur when the corpus luteum fails to break down and instead fills with fluid. They may cause pelvic discomfort, pain or delayed menstruation. They are often seen in early pregnancy.

Other Types of Ovarian Masses

Serous Cystadenoma
These are tumours of the epithelial cells in the ovary.

Mucinous Cystadenoma
These are also tumours of the epithelial cells. They can become huge, taking up lots of space in the pelvis and abdomen.

Endometrioma
These are lumps of endometrial tissue within the ovary, occurring in patients with endometriosis. They can cause pain and disrupt ovulation.

Dermoid Cysts / Germ Cell Tumours
These are benign ovarian tumours. They are *teratomas*, meaning they come from the *germ cells* and may contain various tissue types, such as skin, teeth, hair and bone. They are particularly associated with ovarian torsion.

Sex Cord-Stromal Tumours
These are rare tumours, that can be benign or malignant. They arise from the stroma (connective tissue) or sex cords (embryonic structures associated with the follicles). There are several types, including *Sertoli–Leydig cell tumours* and *granulosa cell tumours*.

Assessment

The key to managing ovarian cysts is to establish whether they are benign or malignant. Take a detailed history and examine for features that may suggest malignancy:

- Abdominal bloating
- Reduce appetite
- Early satiety
- Weight loss
- Urinary symptoms
- Pain
- Ascites
- Lymphadenopathy

Assess for risk factors for ovarian malignancy:

- Age
- Postmenopause
- Increased number of ovulations
- Obesity
- Hormone replacement therapy
- Smoking
- Breastfeeding (protective)
- Family history and BRCA1 and BRCA2 genes

The number of times a woman has ovulated during her life correlates with her risk of ovarian cancer. More ovulations increases the risk of ovarian cancer. Factors that will **reduce** the number of ovulations are:

- Later onset of periods (menarche)
- Early menopause
- Any pregnancies
- Use of the combined contraceptive pill

Blood Tests

Premenopausal women with a *simple ovarian cyst* less than 5cm on *ultrasound* do not need further investigations.

CA125 is the *tumour marker* to remember for ovarian cancer. It contributes to the overall impression of whether an ovarian cyst is related to cancer and forms part of the *risk of malignancy index* (see below).

Women under 40 years with a **complex ovarian mass** require tumour markers for a possible **germ cell tumour**:
- **Lactate dehydrogenase (LDH)**
- **Alpha-fetoprotein (a-FP)**
- **Human chorionic gonadotropin (hCG)**

Causes of Raised CA125

CA125 is a tumour marker for epithelial cell ovarian cancer. It is not very specific, and there are many non-malignant causes of a raised CA125:
- Endometriosis
- Fibroids
- Adenomyosis
- Pelvic infection
- Liver disease
- Pregnancy

Risk of Malignancy Index

The **risk of malignancy index (RMI)** estimates the risk of an ovarian mass being malignant, taking account of three things:
- Menopausal status
- Ultrasound findings
- CA125 level

Management

The **RCOG Green-top guidelines** from 2011 on suspected ovarian masses provides recommendations on managing ovarian cysts. Always check local and national guidelines when deciding how to manage patients, and get advice from an experienced colleague.

Possible **ovarian cancer** (**complex cysts** or **raised CA125**) requires a **two-week wait** referral to a gynaecology oncology specialist.

Possible **dermoid cysts** require referral to a gynaecologist for further investigation and consideration of surgery.

Simple ovarian cysts in **premenopausal women** can be managed based on their size:
- Less than 5cm cysts will almost always resolve within three cycles. They do not require a follow-up scan.
- 5cm to 7cm: Require routine referral to gynaecology and yearly ultrasound monitoring.
- More than 7cm: Consider an MRI scan or surgical evaluation as they can be difficult to characterise with ultrasound.

Cysts in **postmenopausal women** generally require correlation with the CA125 result and referral to a gynaecologist. When there is a raised CA125, this should be a **two-week wait** suspected cancer referral. Simple cysts under 5cm with a normal CA125 may be monitored with an ultrasound every 4 - 6 months.

Persistent or enlarging cysts may require **surgical intervention** (usually with **laparoscopy**). Surgery may involve removing the cyst (**ovarian cystectomy**), possibly along with the affected ovary (**oophorectomy**).

Complications

Consider complications when patients present with acute onset pain. The main complications are:
- **Torsion**
- **Haemorrhage** into the cyst
- **Rupture**, with bleeding into the peritoneum

Meig's Syndrome

Meig's syndrome involves a *triad* of:
- **Ovarian fibroma** (a type of benign ovarian tumour)
- **Pleural effusion**
- **Ascites**

Meig's syndrome typically occurs in older women. Removal of the tumour results in complete resolution of the effusion and ascites.

TOM TIP: It is worth remembering Meig's syndrome for your MCQ exams. Look out for the woman presenting with a pleural effusion and an ovarian mass.

Ovarian Torsion

Ovarian torsion is a condition where the ovary twists in relation to the surrounding connective tissue, fallopian tube and blood supply (the **adnexa**).

Ovarian torsion is usually due to an **ovarian mass** larger than 5cm, such as a **cyst** or a **tumour**. It is more likely to occur with **benign tumours**. It is also more likely to occur during pregnancy.

Ovarian torsion can happen with normal ovaries in younger girls **before menarche** (the first period), when girls have longer **infundibulopelvic ligaments** that can twist more easily.

Twisting of the adnexa and blood supply to the ovary leads to **ischaemia**. If the torsion persists, **necrosis** will occur, and the function of that ovary will be lost. Therefore, ovarian torsion is an **emergency**, where a delay in treatment can have significant consequences. Prompt diagnosis and management is essential.

Presentation

The main presenting feature is **sudden onset severe unilateral pelvic pain**. The pain is constant, gets progressively worse and is associated with **nausea and vomiting**.

The pain is not always severe, and ovarian torsion can take a milder and more prolonged course. Occasionally, the ovary can twist and untwist intermittently, causing pain that comes and goes.

On examination there will be **localised tenderness**. There may be a **palpable mass** in the pelvis, although the absence of a mass does not exclude the diagnosis.

Diagnosis

Pelvic ultrasound is the initial investigation of choice. Transvaginal is ideal, but transabdominal can be used where transvaginal is not possible. It may show the **"whirlpool sign"**, **free fluid** in pelvis and **oedema** of the ovary. Doppler studies may show a lack of blood flow.

The definitive diagnosis is made with **laparoscopic surgery**.

Management

Patients need emergency admission under gynaecology for urgent investigation and management. Depending on the duration and severity of the illness they require **laparoscopic surgery** to either:
- **Untwist** the ovary and fix it in place (**detorsion**)
- **Remove** the affected ovary (**oophorectomy**)

The decision whether to save the ovary or remove it is made during the surgery, based on a visual inspection of the ovary. Laparotomy may be required where there is a large ovarian mass, or malignancy is suspected.

Complications

A delay in treating ovarian torsion can result in loss of function of that ovary. The other ovary can usually compensate, so fertility is not typically affected. Where this is the only functioning ovary, loss of function leads to infertility and menopause.

Where a necrotic ovary is not removed, it may become **infected**, develop an **abscess** and lead to **sepsis**. Additionally it may **rupture**, resulting in **peritonitis** and **adhesions**.

Asherman's Syndrome

Asherman's syndrome is where **adhesions** (sometimes called **synechiae**) form **within the uterus**, following damage to the uterus.

Usually Asherman's syndrome occurs after a pregnancy-related **dilatation and curettage procedure**, for example in the treatment of **retained products of conception** (removing placental tissue left behind after birth). It can also occur after **uterine surgery** (e.g. myomectomy) or **pelvic infection** (e.g. **endometritis**).

Endometrial curettage (scraping) can damage the **basal layer** of the **endometrium**. This damaged tissue may heal abnormally, creating scar tissue (adhesions) connecting areas of the uterus that are generally not connected. There may be adhesions binding the uterine walls together, or within the endocervix, sealing it shut.

These adhesions form physical obstructions and distort the pelvic organs, resulting in menstruation abnormalities, infertility and recurrent miscarriages.

Adhesions may be found incidentally during hysteroscopy. Asymptomatic adhesions are not classified as Asherman's syndrome.

Presentation

Asherman's syndrome typically presents following recent dilatation and curettage, uterine surgery or endometritis with:
- **Secondary amenorrhoea** (absent periods)
- Significantly **lighter periods**
- **Dysmenorrhoea** (painful periods)

It may also present with infertility.

Diagnosis

There are several options for establishing a diagnosis of intrauterine adhesions:
- **Hysteroscopy** is the gold standard investigation, and can involve dissection and treatment of the adhesions
- **Hysterosalpingography**, where contrast is injected into the uterus and imaged with xrays
- **Sonohysterography**, where the uterus is filled with fluid and a pelvic ultrasound is performed
- **MRI scan**

Management

Management is by dissecting the adhesions during hysteroscopy. Reoccurrence of the adhesions after treatment is common.

Cervical Ectropion

Cervical ectropion can also be called **cervical ectopy** or **cervical erosion**. Cervical ectropion occurs when the **columnar epithelium** of the **endocervix** (the canal of the cervix) has extended out to the **ectocervix** (the outer area of the cervix). The lining of the endocervix becomes visible on examination of the cervix using a speculum. This lining has a different appearance to the normal ectocervix.

The cells of the **endocervix** (columnar epithelial cells) are more fragile and prone to trauma. They are more likely to bleed with sexual intercourse. This means cervical ectropion often presents with **postcoital bleeding**.

Cervical ectropion is associated with higher **oestrogen** levels, and therefore, is more common in **younger women**, the **combined contraceptive pill** and **pregnancy**.

Transformation Zone

The **transformation zone** is the border between the **columnar epithelium** of the **endocervix** (the canal), and the **stratified squamous epithelium** of the **ectocervix** (the outer area of the cervix visible on speculum examination). When the transformation zone is located on the **ectocervix**, it is visible during speculum examination as a border between the two epithelial types.

Presentation

Many cervical ectropion are asymptomatic, and they are found incidentally during speculum examination for other reasons, for example, smear tests.

Ectropion may present with **increased vaginal discharge**, **vaginal bleeding** or **dyspareunia** (pain during sex). Intercourse is a common cause of minor trauma to the ectropion, triggering episodes of **postcoital bleeding**.

Examination of the cervix will reveal a well-demarcated border between the redder, velvety **columnar epithelium** extending from the os (opening), and the pale pink **squamous epithelium** of the endocervix. This border is the transformation zone.

TOM TIP: It is worth looking up photographs of cervical ectropion and becoming familiar with the appearance. They are very common to see on speculum examination, and could look alarming the first time you see one. Ectropion are not associated with cervical cancer in any way. It is worth getting familiar with distinguishing them from the appearance of cervical cancer. Always ask about smears, and if in doubt, get a senior opinion and consider referral for colposcopy.

Management

Asymptomatic ectropion require no treatment. Ectropion will typically resolve as the patient gets older, stops the pill or is no longer pregnant. Having a cervical ectropion is not a contraindication to the combined contraceptive pill.

Problematic bleeding is an indication for the treatment of cervical ectropion. Treatment involves **cauterisation** of the ectropion using **silver nitrate** or **cold coagulation** during **colposcopy**.

Nabothian Cysts

Nabothian cysts are fluid-filled cysts often seen on the surface of the cervix. They are also called **nabothian follicles** or **mucinous retention cysts**. They are usually up to 1cm in size, but rarely can be more extensive. They are harmless and unrelated to cervical cancer.

The **columnar epithelium** of the **endocervix** (the canal) produces cervical mucus. When the **squamous epithelium** of the **ectocervix** slightly covers the **mucus-secreting columnar epithelium**, the mucus becomes trapped and forms a cyst. This can happen after **childbirth**, **minor trauma** to the cervix or **cervicitis** secondary to infection.

Presentation

Nabothian cysts are often found incidentally on a speculum examination. They do not typically cause any symptoms. Rarely, when they are very large, they may cause a feeling of fullness in the pelvis.

Nabothian cysts appear as smooth rounded bumps on the cervix, usually near to **os** (opening). They can range in size from 2mm to 30mm, and have a whitish or yellow appearance.

TOM TIP: It is worth becoming familiar with photographs of nabothian cysts. They are relatively common. They can have a raised and discoloured appearance, creating concern when you first see them. With practice, you will be able to identify them correctly, and the woman can be reassured. Getting a senior opinion if there is any doubt creates a feedback loop that helps you confirm your impression and build your confidence in making the correct diagnosis.

Management

Where the diagnosis is clear, women can be reassured, and no treatment is required. They do not cause any harm and often resolve spontaneously.

If the diagnosis is uncertain, women can be referred for **colposcopy** to examine in detail. Occasionally they may be **excised** or **biopsied** to exclude other pathology. Rarely they may be treated during colposcopy to relieve symptoms.

Pelvic Organ Prolapse

Pelvic organ prolapse refers to the descent of pelvic organs into the vagina. Prolapse is the result of weakness and lengthening of the **ligaments** and **muscles** surrounding the **uterus**, **rectum** and **bladder**.

Uterine Prolapse

Uterine prolapse is where the uterus itself descends into the vagina.

Vault Prolapse

Vault prolapse occurs in women that have had a hysterectomy, and no longer have a uterus. The top of the vagina (the vault) descends into the vagina.

Rectocele

Rectoceles are caused by a defect in the **posterior vaginal wall**, allowing the rectum to prolapse forwards into the vagina. Rectoceles are particularly associated with **constipation**. Women can develop **faecal loading** in the part of the rectum that has prolapsed into the vagina. Loading of faeces results in significant **constipation**, **urinary retention** (due to compression on the urethra) and a **palpable lump** in the vagina. Women may use their fingers to press the lump backwards, correcting the anatomical position of the rectum, and allowing them to open their bowels.

Cystocele

Cystoceles are caused by a defect in the **anterior vaginal wall**, allowing the bladder to prolapse backwards into the vagina. Prolapse of the urethra is also possible (**urethrocele**). Prolapse of both the bladder and the urethra is called a **cystourethrocele**.

Risk Factors

Pelvic organ prolapse is the result of weak and stretched muscles and ligaments. The factors that can contribute to this include:
- Multiple vaginal deliveries
- Instrumental, prolonged or traumatic delivery
- Advanced age and postmenopause
- Obesity
- Chronic respiratory disease causing coughing
- Chronic constipation causing straining

Presentation

Typical presenting symptoms are:
- A feeling of "something coming down" in the vagina
- A dragging or heavy sensation in the pelvis
- Urinary symptoms, such as incontinence, urgency, frequency, weak stream and retention
- Bowel symptoms, such as constipation, incontinence and urgency
- Sexual dysfunction, such as pain, altered sensation and reduced enjoyment

Women may have identified a lump or mass in the vagina, and often will already be pushing it back up themselves. They may notice the prolapse will become worse on straining or bearing down.

Examination

Ideally, the patient should empty their bladder and bowel before examination of a prolapse. When examining for pelvic organ prolapse, various positions may be attempted, including the **dorsal** and **left lateral** position.

A **Sim's speculum** is a U-shaped, single-bladed speculum that can be used to support the anterior or posterior vaginal wall while the other vaginal walls are examined. It is held on the anterior wall to examine for a rectocele, and the posterior wall for a cystocele.

The woman can be asked to cough or "bear down" to assess the full descent of the prolapse.

Grades of Uterine Prolapse

The severity of a uterine prolapse can be graded using the **pelvic organ prolapse quantification** (**POP-Q**) system:
- Grade 0: Normal
- Grade 1: The lowest part is more than 1cm above the introitus
- Grade 2: The lowest part is within 1cm of the introitus (above or below)
- Grade 3: The lowest part is more than 1cm below the introitus, but not fully descended
- Grade 4: Full descent with eversion of the vagina

A prolapse extending beyond the introitus can be referred to as **uterine procidentia**.

Management

There are three options for management:
1. Conservative management
2. Vaginal pessary
3. Surgery

Conservative management is appropriate for women that are able to cope with mild symptoms, do not tolerate pessaries or are not suitable for surgery. Conservative management involves:
- **Physiotherapy** (pelvic floor exercises)
- **Weight loss**
- **Lifestyle changes** for associated stress incontinence, such as reduced caffeine intake and incontinence pads
- **Treatment of related symptoms**, such as treating stress incontinence with anticholinergic mediations
- **Vaginal oestrogen cream**

Vaginal pessaries are inserted into the vagina to provide extra support to the pelvic organs. They can create a significant improvement in symptoms and can easily be removed and replaced if they cause any problems. There are many types of pessary:
- **Ring** pessaries are a ring shape, and sit around the cervix holding the uterus up
- **Shelf** and **Gellhorn** pessaries consist of a flat disc with a stem, that sits below the uterus with the stem pointing downwards
- **Cube** pessaries are a cube shape
- **Donut** pessaries consist of a thick ring, similar to a doughnut
- **Hodge** pessaries are almost rectangular. One side is hooked around the posterior aspect of the cervix and the other extends into the vagina.

Women often have to try a few types of pessary before finding the correct comfort and symptom relief. Pessaries should be removed and cleaned or changed periodically (e.g. every four months). They can cause vaginal irritation and erosion over time. **Oestrogen cream** helps protect the vaginal walls from irritation.

Surgery is the definitive option for treating a pelvic organ prolapse. It is essential to consider the risks and benefits of any operation for each individual, taking into account any co-morbidities. There are many methods for surgical correction of a prolapse, including hysterectomy. Surgery can be very successful in correcting the problem. Possible complications of pelvic organ prolapse surgery include:
- Pain, bleeding, infection, DVT and risk of anaesthetic
- Damage to the bladder or bowel
- Recurrence of the prolapse
- Altered experience of sex

Mesh repairs have been the subject of a lot of controversy over recent years. Mesh repairs involve inserting a plastic mesh to support the pelvic organs. After review, NICE recommend that mesh procedures should be avoided entirely. Potential complications associated with mesh repairs are:
- Chronic pain
- Altered sensation
- Dyspareunia (painful sex) for the women or her partner
- Abnormal bleeding
- Urinary or bowel problems

Women presenting with possible complications of mesh repair should be referred to a specialist for assessment and management.

Urinary Incontinence

Urinary incontinence refers to the loss of control of urination. There are two types of urinary incontinence, **urge incontinence** and **stress incontinence**. Establishing the type of incontinence is essential, as this will determine the management.

Urge Incontinence

Urge incontinence is caused by **overactivity** of the **detrusor muscle** of the bladder. Urge incontinence is also known as **overactive bladder**. The typical description is of suddenly feeling the urge to pass urine, having to rush to the bathroom and not arriving before urination occurs. Women with urge incontinence are very conscious about always having access to a toilet, and may avoid activities or places where they may not have easy access. This can have a significant impact on their **quality of life**, and stop them doing work and leisure activities.

Stress Incontinence

The **pelvic floor** consists of a sling of muscles that support the contents of the pelvic. There are three canals through the centre of the female pelvic floor: the **urethral**, **vaginal** and **rectal canals**. When the muscles of the pelvic floor are weak, the canals become lax, and the organs are poorly supported within the pelvis.

Stress incontinence is due to weakness of the **pelvic floor** and **sphincter muscles**. This allows urine to leak at times of increased pressure on the bladder. The typical description of stress incontinence is urinary leakage when laughing, coughing or surprised.

Mixed Incontinence

Mixed incontinence refers to a combination of **urge incontinence** and **stress incontinence**. It is crucial to identify which of the two is having the more significant impact and address this first.

Overflow Incontinence

Overflow incontinence can occur when there is **chronic urinary retention** due to an **obstruction** to the **outflow** of urine. Chronic urinary retention results in an overflow of urine, and the incontinence occurs without the urge to pass urine.

Overflow incontinence can occur with:
- **Anticholinergic medications**
- **Fibroids**
- **Pelvic tumours**
- **Neurological conditions** such as **multiple sclerosis**, **diabetic neuropathy** and **spinal cord injuries**

Overflow incontinence is more common in men, and rare in women. Women with suspected overflow incontinence should be referred for **urodynamic testing** and specialist management.

Risk Factors for Urinary Incontinence

- Increased age
- Postmenopause
- Increase BMI
- Previous pregnancies and vaginal deliveries
- Pelvic organ prolapse
- Pelvic floor surgery
- Neurological conditions, such as multiple sclerosis
- Cognitive impairment and dementia

Assessment

A **medical history** should distinguish between the types of incontinence. Try to differentiate between urinary leakage with coughing or sneezing (**stress incontinence**), and incontinence due to a sudden urge to pass urine with loss of control on the way to the toilet (**urge incontinence**).

Assess for **modifiable lifestyle factors** that can contribute to symptoms:
- Caffeine consumption
- Alcohol consumption
- Medications
- Body mass index (BMI)

Assess the **severity** by asking about:
- Frequency of urination
- Frequency of incontinence
- Nighttime urination
- Use of pads and changes of clothing

Examination should assess the **pelvic tone** and examine for:
- Pelvic organ prolapse
- Atrophic vaginitis
- Urethral diverticulum
- Pelvic masses

During the examination, ask the patient to cough and watch for leakage from the urethra.

The strength of the pelvic muscle contractions can be assessed during a **bimanual examination** by asking the woman to squeeze against the examining fingers. This can be graded using the **modified Oxford grading system**:
- Grade 0: No contraction
- Grade 1: Faint contraction
- Grade 2: Weak contraction
- Grade 3: Moderate contraction with some resistance
- Grade 4: Good contraction with resistance
- Grade 5: Strong contraction, a firm squeeze and drawing inwards of the examining fingers

Investigations

A bladder diary should be completed, tracking fluid intake and episodes of urination and incontinence over at least three days. There should be a mix of work and leisure days covered in the bladder diary.

Urine dipstick testing should be performed to assess for infection, microscopic haematuria and other pathology.

Post-void residual bladder volume should be measured using a bladder scan to assess for incomplete emptying.

Urodynamic testing can be used to investigate patients with urge incontinence not responding to first-line medical treatments, difficulties urinating, urinary retention, previous surgery or an unclear diagnosis. It is not always required where the diagnosis is possible based on the history and examination.

Urodynamic Tests

Urodynamic testing is a way of objectively assessing the presence and severity of urinary symptoms. Patients need to stop taking any **anticholinergic** and bladder related medications around five days before the tests.

A thin catheter is inserted into the bladder, and another into the rectum. These two catheters measure the pressure in the bladder and rectum for comparison. The bladder is filled with liquid, and various outcome measures are taken:
- **Cystometry** measures the detrusor muscle contraction and pressure
- **Uroflowmetry** measures the flow rate
- **Leak point pressure** is the point at which the bladder pressure results in leakage of urine. The patient is asked to cough, move or jump when the bladder is filled to various capacities. This assesses for stress incontinence.
- **Post-void residual bladder volume** tests for incomplete emptying of the bladder
- **Video urodynamic testing** involves filling the bladder with contrast and taking xray images as the bladder is emptied. This is only performed where necessary and not a routine part of urodynamic testing.

Management

The information here is adapted from the NICE guidelines from 2019 on urinary incontinence. Always check local and national guidelines before treating patients.

The first step is to distinguish between urge and stress incontinence, as this dictates the management.

Patients are usually managed in primary care initially and referred to a specialist MDT for further management where there are concerning features or an inadequate response to first-line treatment.

Management of Stress Incontinence

Management of stress incontinence involves:
- Avoiding caffeine, diuretics and overfilling of the bladder
- Avoid excessive or restricted fluid intake
- Weight loss (if appropriate)
- **Supervised pelvic floor exercises** for at least three months before considering surgery
- **Surgery**
- **Duloxetine** is an SNRI antidepressant used second line where surgery is less preferred

Pelvic floor exercises are used to strengthen the muscles of the pelvic floor. They increase the tone and improve the support for the bladder and bowel. Pelvic floor exercises should be supervised by an appropriate professional, such as a specialist nurse or physiotherapist. Women should aim for at least eight contractions, three times daily.

Surgical options to treat stress incontinence include:
- **Tension-free vaginal tape** (TVT) procedures involve a mesh sling looped under the urethra and up behind the pubic symphysis to the abdominal wall. This supports the urethra, reducing stress incontinence.
- **Autologous sling procedures** work similarly to TVT procedures but a strip of fascia from the patient's abdominal wall is used rather than tape
- **Colposuspension** involves stitches connecting the anterior vaginal wall and the pubic symphysis, around the urethra, pulling the vaginal wall forwards and adding support to the urethra
- **Intramural urethral bulking** involves injections around the urethra to reduce the diameter and add support

Where the stress incontinence is caused by a neurological disorder or first line surgical methods have failed, specialist centres may offer an operation to create an **artificial urinary sphincter**. This involves a pump inserted into the labia that inflates and deflates a cuff around the urethra, allowing women to control their continence manually.

Management of Urge Incontinence

Management of urge incontinence and overactive bladder involves:
- **Bladder retraining** (gradually increasing the time between voiding) for at least six weeks is first-line
- **Anticholinergic medication**, for example, oxybutynin, tolterodine and solifenacin
- **Mirabegron** is an alternative to anticholinergic medications
- **Invasive procedures** where medical treatment fails

Anticholinergic medications need to be used carefully, as they have **anticholinergic side effects**. These include dry mouth, dry eyes, urinary retention, constipation and postural hypotension. Importantly they can also lead to a **cognitive decline**, **memory problems** and worsening of **dementia**, which can be very problematic in older, more frail patients.

Mirabegron is used as an alternative medical treatment for urge incontinence, and has less **anticholinergic effects**. However, it is worth noting that mirabegron is **contraindicated** in **uncontrolled hypertension**. Blood pressure needs to be monitored regularly during treatment. It works as a **beta-3 agonist**, stimulating the **sympathetic nervous system**, leading to **raised blood pressure**. This can lead to **hypertensive crisis** and an increased risk of TIA and stroke.

Invasive options for an overactive bladder that has failed to respond to retraining and medical management include:
- **Botulinum toxin type A** injection into the bladder wall
- **Percutaneous sacral nerve stimulation** involves implanting a device in the back that stimulates the sacral nerves
- **Augmentation cystoplasty** involves using bowel tissue to enlarge the bladder
- **Urinary diversion** involves redirecting urinary flow to a urostomy on the abdomen

Atrophic Vaginitis

Atrophic vaginitis refers to **dryness** and **atrophy** of the vaginal mucosa related to a lack of **oestrogen**. Atrophic vaginitis can also be referred to as **genitourinary syndrome of menopause**. It occurs in women from menopause onwards.

The **epithelial lining** of the vagina and urinary tract responds to oestrogen by becoming thicker, more elastic and producing secretions. As women enter the menopause, oestrogen levels fall, resulting in the mucosa becoming **thinner**, **less elastic** and more **dry**. The tissue is more prone to **inflammation**. There are also changes in the **vaginal pH** and **microbial flora** that can contribute to localised infections.

Oestrogen also helps maintain healthy **connective tissue** around the pelvic organs, and a lack of oestrogen can contribute to **pelvic organ prolapse** and **stress incontinence**.

Presentation

Atrophic vaginitis presents in postmenopausal women with symptoms of:
- Itching
- Dryness
- Dyspareunia (discomfort or pain during sex)
- Bleeding due to localised inflammation

You should also consider atrophic vaginitis in older women presenting with **recurrent urinary tract infections, stress incontinence** and **pelvic organ prolapse**. Treatment with topical oestrogen where appropriate may improve the symptoms of these conditions.

It is worth asking about symptoms of vaginal dryness and discomfort, as women will often be reluctant to bring it up during a consultation. It is straightforward to treat and can make a big difference to their quality of life.

Examination

Examination of the labia and vagina will demonstrate:
- Pale mucosa
- Thin skin
- Reduced skin folds
- Erythema and inflammation
- Dryness
- Sparse pubic hair

Management

Vaginal lubricants can help symptoms of dryness. Examples include **Sylk**, **Replens** and **YES**.

Topical oestrogen can make a big difference in symptoms. Options include:
- **Estriol cream**, applied using an applicator (syringe) at bedtime
- **Estriol pessaries**, inserted at bedtime
- **Estradiol tablets** (**Vagifem**), once daily
- **Estradiol ring** (**Estring**), replaced every three months

Topical oestrogen shares many **contraindications** with **systemic HRT**, such as **breast cancer**, **angina** and **venous thromboembolism**. It is unclear whether long term use of topical oestrogen increases the risk of endometrial hyperplasia and endometrial cancer. Women should be monitored at least annually, with a view of stopping treatment when possible.

Bartholin's Cyst

The **Bartholin's glands** are a pair glands located either side of the posterior part of the **vaginal introitus** (the vaginal opening). They are usually pea-sized and not palpable. They produce mucus to help with vaginal lubrication.

When the ducts become blocked, the Bartholin's glands can swell and become tender, causing a **Bartholin's cyst**. The swelling is typically unilateral and forms a fluid-filled cyst between 1 - 4 cm.

Cysts can become infected, forming a **Bartholin's abscess**. A Bartholin's abscess will be hot, tender, red and potentially draining pus.

A diagnosis of a Bartholin's cyst or abscess is made clinically with a history and examination.

Management

Bartholin's cysts will usually resolve with simple treatment such as good hygiene, analgesia and warm compresses. Incision is generally avoided, as the cyst will often reoccur. A **biopsy** may be required if **vulval malignancy** needs to be excluded (particularly in women over 40 years).

A **Bartholin's abscess** will require **antibiotics**. A **swab** of pus or fluid from the abscess can be taken to **culture** the infective organism and check the **antibiotic sensitivities**. *E. coli* is the most common cause. Send specific swabs for **chlamydia** and **gonorrhoea**.

Surgical interventions may be required to treat a Bartholin's abscess. There are two options for surgical management:
- **Word catheter** (Bartholin's gland balloon) - requires local anaesthetic
- **Marsupialisation** - requires general anaesthetic

A **Word catheter** is a small rubber tube with a balloon on the end. The procedure may be performed by an appropriately experienced person in a treatment room, rather than a theatre. **Local anaesthetic** is used to numb the area. An incision is made, and any pus is drained from the abscess. The Word catheter is inserted into the abscess space, and inflated up to 3 ml with saline. The balloon fills the space and keeps the catheter in place. Fluid can drain around the catheter, preventing a cyst or abscess reoccurring. The tissue heals around the catheter, leaving a permanent hole. The catheter can be deflated and carefully removed at a later date, once epithelisation of the hole has occurred.

Marsupialisation involves a **general anaesthetic** in a **surgical theatre**. An incision is made, and the abscess is drained. The sides of the abscess are sutured open. Suturing the abscess open allows continuous drainage of the area and prevents recurrence of the cyst or abscess.

Lichen Sclerosus

Lichen sclerosus is a **chronic inflammatory** skin condition that presents with patches of shiny, "**porcelain-white**" skin. It commonly affects the **labia**, **perineum** and **perianal** skin in women. It can affect other areas, such as the axilla and thighs. It can also affect men, typically on the **foreskin** and **glans** of the penis.

Lichen sclerosus is thought to be an **autoimmune condition**. It is associated with other autoimmune diseases, such as **type 1 diabetes**, **alopecia**, **hypothyroid** and **vitiligo**.

The diagnosis of lichen sclerosus is usually made clinically, based on the history and examination findings. Where there is doubt, a **vulval biopsy** can confirm the diagnosis.

Lichen

Lichen sclerosis may be confused with other conditions that include "**lichen**" in the name. Lichen refers to a flat eruption that spreads. It is important not to get lichen sclerosus confused with **lichen simplex** or **lichen planus**.

Lichen simplex is chronic inflammation and irritation caused by repeated scratching and rubbing of an area of skin. This presents with excoriations, plaques, scaling and thickened skin.

Lichen planus is an autoimmune condition that causes localised chronic inflammation with shiny, purplish, flat-topped, raised areas with white lines across the surface called **Wickham's striae**.

Presentation

The typical presentation in your exams is a woman aged 45 - 60 years complaining of **vulval itching** and **skin changes** in the vulva. The condition may be **asymptomatic**, or present with several symptoms:

- Itching
- Soreness and pain, possibly worse at night
- Skin tightness
- Painful sex (superficial dyspareunia)
- Erosions
- Fissures

The **Koebner phenomenon** refers to when the signs and symptoms are made worse by friction to the skin. This occurs with lichen sclerosus. It can be made worse by tight underwear that rubs the skin, urinary incontinence and scratching.

Appearance

Changes affect the labia, perianal and perineal skin. There can be associated fissures, cracks, erosions or haemorrhages under the skin. The affected skin appears:

- "Porcelain-white" in colour
- Shiny
- Tight
- Thin
- Slightly raised
- There may be papules or plaques

Management

The management here is based on the 2018 guidelines from the **British Association of Dermatologists**. Lichen sclerosis cannot be cured, but the symptoms can be effectively controlled. Lichen sclerosus is usually managed and followed up every 3 - 6 months by an experienced gynaecologist or dermatologist.

Potent topical steroids are the mainstay of treatment. The typical choice is **clobetasol propionate 0.05% (Dermovate)**. Steroids are used long term to control the symptoms of the condition. They also seem to reduce the risk of malignancy.

Steroids are initially used once a day for four weeks, then gradually reduced in frequency every four weeks to alternate days, then twice weekly. When the condition flares patients can go back to using topical steroids daily until they achieve good control. A 30g tube should last at least three months.

Emollients should be used regularly, both with steroids initially and then as part of maintenance.

Complications

The critical complication to remember is a 5% risk of developing **squamous cell carcinoma** of the **vulva**.

Other complications include:
- Pain and discomfort
- Sexual dysfunction
- Bleeding
- Narrowing of the vaginal or urethral openings

Female Genital Mutilation

Female genital mutilation (**FGM**) involves surgically changing the genitals of a female for non-medical reasons. FGM is a cultural practice that usually occurs in girls before puberty. It is a form of **child abuse** and a **safeguarding** issue.

Female genital mutilation is illegal as stated in the **Female Genital Mutilation Act 2003**, and there is a legal requirement for healthcare professionals to report cases of FGM to the police.

Epidemiology

UNICEF provides information and data on the epidemiology of FGM. FGM is a common cultural practice in many African countries. Somalia has the highest levels of FGM in any country. Other countries with high rates are Ethiopia, Sudan and Eritrea. It also occurs in Yemen, Kurdistan, Indonesia and various parts of South and Western Asia.

Types

There are four types of female genital mutilation:
- **Type 1**: Removal of part or all of the clitoris.
- **Type 2**: Removal of part or all of the clitoris and labia minora. The labia majora may also be removed.
- **Type 3**: Narrowing or closing the vaginal orifice (**infibulation**).
- **Type 4**: All other unnecessary procedures to the female genitalia.

Identifying Cases

It is important to recognise risk factors for FGM to identify and ideally prevent cases from occurring. Two key risk factors to bear in mind are coming from a community that practise FGM and having relatives affected by FGM.

There are scenarios where it is worth considering the risk of FGM:
- Pregnant women with FGM with a possible female child
- Siblings or daughters of women or girls affected by FGM
- Extended trips with infants or children to areas where FGM is practised
- Women that decline examination or cervical screening
- New patients from communities that practise FGM

Women may also present with the complications of FGM.

Complications

Immediate complications include:
- Pain
- Bleeding
- Infection
- Swelling
- Urinary retention
- Urethral damage and incontinence

Long term complications include:
- Vaginal infections, such as bacterial vaginosis
- Pelvic infections
- Urinary tract infections
- **Dysmenorrhea** (painful menstruation)
- Sexual dysfunction and **dyspareunia** (painful sex)
- Infertility and pregnancy-related complications
- Significant psychological issues and depression
- Reduced engagement with healthcare and screening

Management

It is essential to educate patients and relatives that FGM is illegal in the UK. Discuss the health consequences of FGM.

It is **mandatory** to report all cases of FGM in patients **under 18** to the police.

Other services should also be contacted:
- Social services and safeguarding
- Paediatrics
- Specialist gynaecology or FGM services
- Counselling

In patients over 18, there needs to be careful consideration about whether to report cases to the police or social services. The RCOG recommends using a risk assessment tool to tackle this issue (available on the gov.uk website). The risk assessment includes considering whether the patient has female relatives that may be at risk. If the unborn child of a pregnant woman affected by FGM is considered to be at risk, a referral should be made.

A **de-infibulation** surgical procedure may be performed by a specialist in FGM in cases of type 3 FGM. This aims to correct the narrowing or closure of the vaginal orifice, improve symptoms and try to restore normal function.

Re-infibulation (re-closure of the vaginal orifice) may be requested by women after childbirth. However, performing this procedure is illegal.

Congenital Structural Abnormalities

Congenital structural abnormalities of the reproductive tract are caused by abnormal development of the pelvic organs prior to birth. This can lead to menstrual, sexual and reproductive problems. These abnormalities may be the result of faulty genes, or occur randomly in otherwise healthy individuals. This section covers some of the key congenital structural abnormalities that you may encounter in your exams and career.

Basic Embryological Development

The **upper vagina**, **cervix**, **uterus** and **fallopian tubes** develop from the **paramesonephric ducts** (**Mullerian ducts**). These are a pair of passageways along the outside of the urogenital region that fuse and mature to become the uterus, fallopian tubes, cervix and upper third of the vagina. Errors in their development lead to congenital structural abnormalities in the female pelvic organs. In a male fetus, **anti-Mullerian hormone** is produced, which suppresses the growth of the paramesonephric ducts, causing them to disappear.

TOM TIP: If you remember one thing about the embryology of the female reproductive system, remember the Mullerian ducts. Medical school exams are unlikely to test your knowledge of the embryology of the female reproductive system in detail (unless the exam is specific to that topic). However, they may refer to a congenital structural abnormality and ask what structure in the fetus this relates to. The answer is the Mullerian ducts. Equally, they may ask why males do not develop a uterus, and the answer is anti-Mullerian hormone.

Bicornuate Uterus

A bicornuate uterus is where there are two "horns" to the uterus, giving the uterus a heart-shaped appearance. It can be diagnosed on a pelvic ultrasound scan. A bicornuate uterus may be associated with adverse pregnancy outcomes. However, successful pregnancies are generally expected. In most cases, no specific management is required.

Typical complications include:
- Miscarriage
- Premature birth
- Malpresentation

Imperforate Hymen

Imperforate hymen is where the hymen at the entrance of the vagina is fully formed, without an opening.

Imperforate hymen may be discovered when the girl starts to menstruate, and the menses are sealed in the vagina. This causes cyclical pelvic pain and cramping that would ordinarily be associated with menstruation, but without any vaginal bleeding.

An imperforate hymen can be diagnosed during a clinical examination. Treatment is with surgical incision to create an opening in the hymen.

Theoretically, if an imperforate hymen is not treated **retrograde menstruation** could occur leading to **endometriosis**.

Transverse Vaginal Septae

Transverse vaginal septae are caused by an error in development, where a **septum** (wall) forms **transversely** across the vagina. This septum can either be **perforate** (with a hole) or **imperforate** (completely sealed). Where it is perforate, girls will still menstruate, but can have difficulty with intercourse or tampon use. Where it is imperforate, it will present similarly to an imperforate hymen with cyclical pelvic symptoms without menstruation. Vaginal septae can lead to infertility and pregnancy-related complications.

Diagnosis is by examination, ultrasound or MRI. Treatment is with surgical correction. The main complications of surgery are **vaginal stenosis** and **recurrence** of the septae.

Vaginal Hypoplasia and Agenesis

Vaginal hypoplasia refers to an abnormally small vagina. **Vaginal agenesis** refers to an absent vagina. These occur due to failure of the **Mullerian ducts** to properly develop, and may be associated with an absent uterus and cervix.

The ovaries are usually unaffected, leading to normal female sex hormones. The exception to this is with **androgen insensitivity syndrome**, where there are testes rather than ovaries.

Management may involve the use of a **vaginal dilator** over a prolonged period to create an adequate vaginal size. Alternatively, vaginal surgery may be necessary.

Androgen Insensitivity Syndrome

Androgen insensitivity syndrome is a condition where cells are unable to respond to **androgen hormones** due to a lack of **androgen receptors**. It is an **X-linked recessive** genetic condition, caused by a mutation in the **androgen receptor gene** on the **X chromosome**. Extra androgens are converted into oestrogen, resulting in **female secondary sexual characteristics**. It was previously known as **testicular feminisation syndrome**.

Patients with androgen insensitivity syndrome are **genetically male**, with **XY sex chromosome**. However, the absent response to testosterone and the conversion of additional androgens to **oestrogen** result in a **female phenotype** externally. Typical male sexual characteristics do not develop, and patients have normal female external genitalia and breast tissue.

Patients have **testes** in the abdomen or inguinal canal, and absence of a **uterus, upper vagina, cervix, fallopian tubes** and **ovaries**. The female internal organs do not develop because the **testes** produce **anti-Müllerian hormone**, which prevents males from developing an **upper vagina**, **uterus**, **cervix** and **fallopian tubes**.

The insensitivity to androgens also results in a lack of pubic hair, facial hair and male type muscle development. Patients tend to be slightly taller than the female average. Patients are infertile, and there is an increased risk of testicular cancer unless the testes are removed.

This section mainly covers **complete androgen insensitivity syndrome**. There is also a condition called **partial androgen insensitivity syndrome**, where the cells have a partial response to androgens. This presents with more ambiguous signs and symptoms, such as a micropenis or clitoromegaly, bifid scrotum, hypospadias and diminished male characteristics.

Presentation

Androgen insensitivity syndrome often presents in infancy with **inguinal hernias** that contain testes. Alternatively, it presents at puberty with **primary amenorrhoea**. The results of hormone tests are:
- Raised LH
- Normal or raised FSH
- Normal or raised testosterone levels (for a male)
- Raised oestrogen levels (for a male)

Management

Management is coordinated by a specialist MDT, involving paediatrics, gynaecology, urology, endocrinology and clinical psychology. Medical input involves:
- **Bilateral orchidectomy** (removal of the testes) to avoid testicular tumours
- **Oestrogen therapy**
- **Vaginal dilators** or **vaginal surgery** can be used to create an adequate vaginal length

Generally, patients are raised as female, but this is sensitive and tailored to the individual. They are offered support and counselling to help them understand the condition and promote their psychological, social and sexual wellbeing.

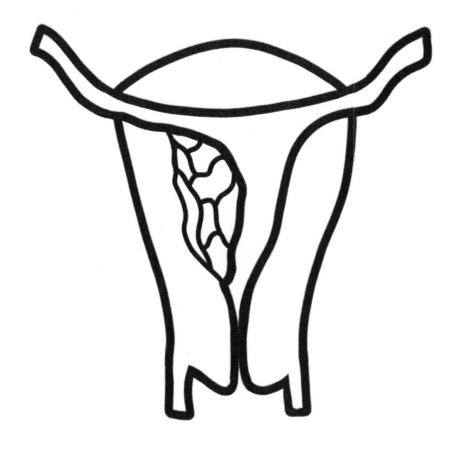

CANCER

3.1	Cervical Cancer	71
3.2	Endometrial Cancer	75
3.3	Ovarian Cancer	78
3.4	Vulval Cancer	80

Cervical Cancer

Cancer of the cervix tends to affect younger women, peaking in the reproductive years. 80% of cervical cancers are **squamous cell carcinoma**. **Adenocarcinoma** is the next most common type. Very rarely there are other types, such as small cell cancer.

Cervical cancer is strongly associated with **human papillomavirus**. Children aged 12 - 13 years are vaccinated against certain strains of HPV to reduce the risk of cervical cancer.

Cervical screening with **smear tests** is used to screen for precancerous and cancerous changes to the cells of the cervix. Early detection of precancerous changes enables prompt treatment to prevent the development of cervical cancer.

Human Papilloma Virus

The most common cause of cervical cancer is infection with **human papillomavirus** (**HPV**). HPV is also associated with anal, vulval, vaginal, penile, mouth and throat cancers. HPV is primarily a **sexually transmitted infection**.

There are over 100 strains of HPV. The important ones to remember are **type 16** and **18**, as these are responsible for around 70% of cervical cancers and also the strains targeted with the HPV vaccine. There is no treatment for infection with HPV. Most cases resolve spontaneously within two years, while some will persist.

P53 and **pRb** are **tumour suppressor genes**. They have a role in suppressing cancers from developing. **HPV** produces two proteins (**E6** and **E7**) that **inhibit** these **tumour suppressor genes**. The **E6 protein** inhibits **p53**, and the **E7 protein** inhibits **pRb**. Therefore, HPV promotes the development of cancer by inhibiting tumour suppressor genes.

Risk Factors

You can think of the risk factors for cervical cancer in terms of:
- Increased risk of catching HPV
- Later detection of precancerous and cancerous changes (non-engagement with screening)
- Other risk factors

Increased risk of catching HPV occurs with:
- Early sexual activity
- Increased number of sexual partners
- Sexual partners who have had more partners
- Not using condoms

Non-engagement with cervical screening is a significant risk factor. Many cases of cervical cancer are preventable with early detection and treatment of precancerous changes.

Other risk factors are:
- **Smoking**
- **HIV** (patients with HIV are offered yearly smear tests)
- **Combined contraceptive pill** use for more than five years
- Increased number of **full-term pregnancies**
- **Family history**
- Exposure to **diethylstilbestrol** during fetal development (this was previously used to prevent miscarriages before 1971)

TOM TIP: When you are performing a history in your exams and considering cancer, always ask about risk factors to show your examiners you are assessing that patient's risk of having cancer. Ask about attendance to smears, number of sexual partners, family history and smoking.

Presentation

Cervical cancer may be detected during cervical smears in otherwise **asymptomatic** women.

The presenting symptoms that should make you consider cervical cancer as a differential are:
- Abnormal vaginal bleeding (**intermenstrual**, **postcoital** or **post-menopausal bleeding**)
- Abnormal vaginal discharge
- Pelvic pain
- Dyspareunia (pain or discomfort with sex)

These symptoms are **non-specific**, and in most cases, not caused by cervical cancer. The next step is to examine the cervix with a speculum. During examination, swabs can be taken to exclude infection.

Where there is an abnormal appearance of the cervix suggestive of cancer, an **urgent cancer referral** for **colposcopy** should be made to assess further. Appearances that may suggest cervical cancer are:
- Ulceration
- Inflammation
- Bleeding
- Visible tumour

The **NICE Clinical Knowledge Summaries** (2017) recommend against unscheduled cervical screening with a smear test. They also advise against using the result of cervical screening to exclude cervical cancer where it is suspected for another reason, even if the smear result was normal.

Cervical Intraepithelial Neoplasia

Cervical intraepithelial neoplasia (**CIN**) is a grading system for the level of **dysplasia** (premalignant change) in the cells of the cervix. CIN is diagnosed at **colposcopy** (**not** with cervical screening). The grades are:
- **CIN I**: mild dysplasia, affecting 1/3 the thickness of the epithelial layer, likely to return to normal without treatment
- **CIN II**: moderate dysplasia, affecting 2/3 the thickness of the epithelial layer, likely to progress to cancer if untreated
- **CIN III**: severe dysplasia, very likely to progress to cancer if untreated

CIN III is sometimes called **cervical carcinoma in situ**.

TOM TIP: Try not to get mixed up between dysplasia found during colposcopy and dyskaryosis on smear results.

Screening

Screening for cervical cancer aims to pick up precancerous changes in the epithelial cells of the cervix. It involves a cervical **smear test**, performed by a qualified person, often a **practice nurse**. The test consists of a speculum examination and collection of cells from the cervix using a small brush. The cells are deposited from the brush into a preservation fluid. This fluid is transported to a lab where the cells are examined under a microscope for precancerous changes (**dyskaryosis**). This way of transporting the cells is called **liquid-based cytology**.

The samples are initially tested for **high-risk HPV** before the cells are examined. If the HPV test is negative (the person does not have HPV), the cells are not examined, the smear is considered negative, and the woman is returned to the routine screening program.

The cervical screening program involves performing a smear for women (and transgender men that still have a cervix):
- Every three years aged 25 - 49
- Every five years aged 50 - 64

There are some notable exceptions to the program:
- Women with HIV are screened annually
- Women over 65 may request a smear if they have not had one since aged 50
- Women with previous CIN may require additional tests (e.g. test of cure after treatment)
- Certain groups of immunocompromised women may have additional screening (e.g. women on dialysis, cytotoxic drugs or undergoing an organ transplant)
- Pregnant women due a routine smear should wait until 12 weeks post-partum

Cytology results:
- Inadequate
- Normal
- Borderline changes
- Low-grade dyskaryosis
- High-grade dyskaryosis (moderate)
- High-grade dyskaryosis (severe)
- Possible invasive squamous cell carcinoma
- Possible glandular neoplasia

Infections such as **bacterial vaginosis**, **candidiasis** and **trichomoniasis** may be identified and reported on the smear result.

Actinomyces-like organisms are often discovered in women with an **intrauterine device** (coil). These do not require treatment unless they are symptomatic. Where the woman is symptomatic (e.g. pelvic pain or abnormal bleeding), removal of the intrauterine device may be considered.

A summary of the management of smear results based on the **Public Health England guidelines** from 2019 is:
- Inadequate sample - repeat the smear after at least three months
- HPV negative - continue routine screening
- HPV positive with normal cytology - repeat the HPV test after 12 months
- HPV positive with abnormal cytology - refer for colposcopy

Colposcopy

A specialist performs colposcopy. It involves inserting a speculum and using equipment (a **colposcope**) to magnify the cervix. This allows the epithelial lining of the cervix to be examined in detail. During colposcopy, stains such as **acetic acid** and **iodine solution** can be used to differentiate abnormal areas.

Acetic acid causes abnormal cells to appear white. This appearance is described as **acetowhite**. This occurs in cells with an increased **nuclear to cytoplasmic ratio** (more **nuclear material**), such as **cervical intraepithelial neoplasia** and **cervical cancer** cells.

Schiller's iodine test involves using an **iodine solution** to stain the cells of the cervix. Iodine will stain healthy cells a brown colour. Abnormal areas will not stain.

A **punch biopsy** or **large loop excision of the transformational zone** can be performed during the colposcopy procedure to get a tissue sample.

Large Loop Excision of the Transformation Zone (LLETZ)

A large loop excision of the transformation zone (**LLETZ**) procedure is also called a **loop biopsy**. It can be performed with a **local anaesthetic** during a colposcopy procedure. It involves using a loop of wire with electrical current (**diathermy**) to remove abnormal epithelial tissue on the cervix. The electrical current **cauterises** the tissue and stops bleeding.

Bleeding and abnormal discharge can occur for several weeks following a LLETZ procedure. This varies between women. Intercourse and tampon use should be avoided after the procedure to reduce the risk of infection. Depending on the depth of the tissue removed from the cervix, the procedure may increase the risk of **preterm labour**.

Cone Biopsy

A cone biopsy is a treatment for **cervical intraepithelial neoplasia** (**CIN**) and very early-stage cervical cancer. It involves a general anaesthetic. The surgeon removes a cone-shaped piece of the cervix using a scalpel. This sample is sent for histology to assess for malignancy.

The main risks of a cone biopsy are:
- Pain
- Bleeding
- Infection
- Scar formation with **stenosis** of the cervix
- Increased risk of miscarriage and premature labour

Staging

The **International Federation of Gynaecology and Obstetrics** (**FIGO**) staging system is used to stage cervical cancer:
- Stage 1: Confined to the cervix
- Stage 2: Invades the uterus or upper 2/3 of the vagina
- Stage 3: Invades the pelvic wall or lower 1/3 of the vagina
- Stage 4: Invades the bladder, rectum or beyond the pelvis

Management

Management of cervical cancer depends on the stage and the individual situation. The usual treatments are:
- **Cervical intraepithelial neoplasia** and **early-stage 1A**: LLETZ or cone biopsy
- **Stage 1B - 2A**: Radical hysterectomy and removal of local lymph nodes with chemotherapy and radiotherapy
- **Stage 2B - 4A**: Chemotherapy and radiotherapy
- **Stage 4B**: Management may involve a combination of surgery, radiotherapy, chemotherapy and palliative care

The **5-year survival** drops significantly with more advanced cervical cancer, from around 98% with stage 1A to around 15% with stage 4. Early detection makes a significant difference, which is one reason the screening program is so valuable and important.

Pelvic exenteration is an operation that may be used in advanced cervical cancer. It involves removing most or all of the pelvic organs, including the vagina, cervix, uterus, fallopian tubes, ovaries, bladder and rectum. It is a vast operation and has significant implications on quality of life.

Bevacizumab (**Avastin**) is a monoclonal antibody that may be used in combination with other chemotherapies in the treatment of **metastatic** or **recurrent** cervical cancer. It is also used in several other types of cancer. It targets **vascular endothelial growth factor A** (**VEGF-A**), which is responsible for the development of new blood vessels. Therefore, it reduces the development of new blood vessels. You may also come across this medication as a treatment for **wet age-related macular degeneration**, where it is injected directly into the patient's eye to stop new blood vessels forming on the retina.

Human Papillomavirus (HPV) Vaccine

The HPV vaccine is ideally given to girls and boys **before** they become sexually active. The intention is to prevent them contracting and spreading HPV once they become sexually active. The current NHS vaccine is **Gardasil**, which protects against strains 6, 11, 16 and 18:
- Strains 6 and 11 cause **genital warts**
- Strains 16 and 18 cause **cervical cancer**

TOM TIP: A common exam task is to counsel parents about their child receiving the HPV vaccine. They are upset because they believe this implies their daughter or son is sexually promiscuous. Focus on the fact it needs to be given before they become sexually active and that it protects them from cervical cancer and genital warts. HPV is very common and infection is the number one risk factor for cervical cancer.

Endometrial Cancer

Endometrial cancer is cancer of the **endometrium**, the lining of the **uterus**. Around 80% of cases are **adenocarcinoma**. It is an **oestrogen-dependent cancer**, meaning that **oestrogen** stimulates the growth of endometrial cancer cells.

TOM TIP: For your exams, any woman presenting with postmenopausal bleeding has endometrial cancer until proven otherwise. The key risk factors to remember are obesity and diabetes.

Endometrial Hyperplasia

Endometrial hyperplasia is a **precancerous** condition involving thickening of the endometrium. The risk factors, presentation and investigations of endometrial hyperplasia are similar to endometrial cancer. Most cases of endometrial hyperplasia will return to normal over time. Less than 5% go on to become endometrial cancer. There are two types of endometrial hyperplasia to be aware of:
- **Hyperplasia without atypia**
- **Atypical hyperplasia**

Endometrial hyperplasia may be treated by a specialist using **progestogens**, with either:
- **Intrauterine system** (e.g. Mirena coil)
- **Continuous oral progestogens** (e.g. medroxyprogesterone or levonorgestrel)

Risk Factors

You can think of the risk factors for endometrial cancer in relation to the patient's exposure to **unopposed oestrogen**. Unopposed oestrogen refers to oestrogen without progesterone. Unopposed oestrogen stimulates the endometrial cells and increases the risk of endometrial hyperplasia and cancer. The risk endometrial cancer is associated with the amount of unopposed oestrogen the endometrium is exposed to during the patient's life. Situations where there is increased exposure of unopposed oestrogen are:

- Increased age
- Earlier onset of menstruation
- Late menopause
- Oestrogen only hormone replacement therapy
- No or fewer pregnancies
- Obesity
- Polycystic ovarian syndrome
- Tamoxifen

Polycystic ovarian syndrome leads to increased exposure to **unopposed oestrogen** due to a lack of ovulation. Usually, when ovulation occurs, a **corpus luteum** is formed in the ovaries from the ruptured **follicle** that released the egg. It is the **corpus luteum** that produces **progesterone**, providing endometrial protection during the **luteal phase** of the **menstrual cycle** (the second half of the menstrual cycle). Women with polycystic ovarian syndrome are less likely to ovulate and form a corpus luteum. Without developing a corpus luteum during the menstrual cycle, progesterone is not produced, and the endometrial lining has more exposure to unopposed oestrogen. For endometrial protection, women with PCOS should have one of:

- The **combined contraceptive pill**
- An **intrauterine system** (e.g. Mirena coil)
- **Cyclical progestogens** to induce a withdrawal bleed.

Obesity is a crucial risk factor because **adipose tissue** (fat) is a source of **oestrogen**. Adipose tissue is the primary source of oestrogen in **postmenopausal women**. Adipose tissue contains **aromatase**, which is an enzyme that converts **androgens** such as **testosterone** into **oestrogen**. Androgens are produced mainly by the **adrenal glands**. In women with more adipose tissue, and therefore more aromatase enzyme, more of these androgens are converted to oestrogen. This extra oestrogen is **unopposed** in women that are not ovulating (e.g. PCOS or postmenopause), because there is no corpus luteum to produce progesterone.

Tamoxifen has an anti-oestrogenic effect on breast tissue, but an oestrogenic effect on the endometrium. This increases the risk of endometrial cancer.

Additional risk factors not related to unopposed oestrogen are:

- Type 2 diabetes
- Hereditary non-polyposis colorectal cancer (HNPCC) or Lynch syndrome

Type 2 diabetes may increase the risk of endometrial cancer due to the increased production of **insulin**. Insulin may stimulate the endometrial cells and increase the risk of endometrial hyperplasia and cancer. **PCOS** is also associated with **insulin resistance** and increased **insulin production**. Insulin resistance further adds to the risk of endometrial cancer in women with PCOS.

Protective Factors

Protective factors against endometrial cancer include:
- Combined contraceptive pill
- Mirena coil
- Increased pregnancies
- Cigarette smoking

Smoking appears to be protective against endometrial cancer in postmenopausal women by being anti-oestrogenic. Interestingly, it is not protective against other oestrogen dependent cancers, such as breast cancer (where it increases the risk). Smoking may have anti-oestrogenic effects in several ways:

- Oestrogen may be metabolised differently in smokers
- Smokers tend to be leaner, meaning they have less adipose tissue and aromatase enzyme
- Smoking destroys oocytes (eggs), resulting in an earlier menopause

Presentation

The number one presenting symptom of endometrial cancer to remember for your exams is **postmenopausal bleeding**.

Endometrial cancer may also present with:
- Postcoital bleeding
- Intermenstrual bleeding
- Unusually heavy menstrual bleeding
- Abnormal vaginal discharge
- Haematuria
- Anaemia
- Raised platelet count

Referral Criteria

It is worth being familiar with the NICE "***suspected cancer: recognition and referral***" guidelines (2015) concerning all common cancers. The guidelines contain the referral criteria and red flags for each type of cancer, and will help you quickly recognise or exclude red flag criteria.

The referral criteria for a ***2-week-wait*** urgent cancer referral for endometrial cancer is:
- **Postmenopausal bleeding** (more than 12 months after the last menstrual period)

NICE also recommends referral for a ***transvaginal ultrasound*** in women over 55 years with:
- **Unexplained vaginal discharge**
- **Visible haematuria** PLUS *raised platelets*, *anaemia* or *elevated glucose levels*

Investigations

There are three investigations to remember for diagnosing and excluding endometrial cancer:
- ***Transvaginal ultrasound*** for **endometrial thickness** (normal is **less than 4mm** post-menopause)
- ***Pipelle biopsy***, which is highly **sensitive** for endometrial cancer making it useful for excluding cancer
- ***Hysteroscopy*** with endometrial biopsy

A ***pipelle biopsy*** can be taken in the outpatient clinic. It involves a speculum examination and inserting a thin tube (pipelle) through the cervix into the uterus. This small tube fills with a sample of endometrial tissue that can be examined for signs of endometrial hyperplasia or cancer. Pipelle biopsy is a quicker and less invasive alternative to hysteroscopy for excluding cancer in lower-risk women.

Depending on local guidelines, a normal ***transvaginal ultrasound*** (endometrial thickness < 4mm) and normal ***pipelle biopsy*** are sufficient to demonstrate a very low risk of endometrial cancer and discharge the patient.

Stages

The ***International Federation of Gynaecology and Obstetrics*** (**FIGO**) staging system is used to stage endometrial cancer:
- Stage 1: Confined to the uterus
- Stage 2: Invades the cervix
- Stage 3: Invades the ovaries, fallopian tubes, vagina or lymph nodes
- Stage 4: Invades the bladder, rectum or beyond the pelvis

Management

The usual treatment for stage 1 and 2 endometrial cancer is a **total abdominal hysterectomy with bilateral salpingo-oophorectomy**, also known as a **TAH and BSO** (removal of uterus, cervix and adnexa).

Other treatment options depending on the individual presentation include:
- **Radical hysterectomy** involves also removing the pelvic lymph nodes, surrounding tissues and top of the vagina
- Radiotherapy
- Chemotherapy
- **Progesterone** may be used as a hormonal treatment to slow the progression of the cancer

Ovarian Cancer

Ovarian cancer refers to cancer of the ovaries. Ovarian cancer often presents late due to the **non-specific symptoms**, resulting in a worse prognosis. More than 70% of patients with ovarian cancer present after it has spread beyond the pelvis.

Types of Ovarian Cancer

Epithelial Cell Tumours
Epithelial cell tumours (tumours arising from the **epithelial cells** of the ovary) are the most common type. Subtypes of epithelial cell tumours include:
- **Serous tumours** (the most common)
- Endometrioid carcinomas
- Clear cell tumours
- Mucinous tumours
- Undifferentiated tumours

Dermoid Cysts / Germ Cell Tumours
These are benign ovarian tumours. They are **teratomas**, meaning they come from the **germ cells**. They may contain various tissue types, such as skin, teeth, hair and bone. They are particularly associated with **ovarian torsion**. Germ cell tumours may cause raised **alpha-fetoprotein (α-FP)** and **human chorionic gonadotrophin (hCG)**.

Sex Cord-Stromal Tumours
These are rare tumours, that can be benign or malignant. They arise from the **stroma** (connective tissue) or **sex cords** (embryonic structures associated with the follicles). There are several types, including **Sertoli-Leydig cell tumours** and **granulosa cell tumours**.

Metastasis
Ovarian tumours may be due to metastasis from a cancer elsewhere. A **Krukenberg tumour** refers to a metastasis in the ovary, usually from a **gastrointestinal tract cancer**, particularly the stomach. **Krukenberg tumours** have characteristic **"signet-ring"** cells on histology, which look like signet rings under a microscopy.

Risk factors

- Age (peaks age 60)
- BRCA1 and BRCA2 genes (consider the family history)
- Increased number of ovulations
- Obesity
- Smoking
- Recurrent use of clomifene

Factors that increase the number of ovulations, increase the risk of ovarian cancer. These include:
- Early onset of periods
- Late menopause
- No pregnancies

Protective Factors

Having a higher number of lifetime ovulations increases the risk of ovarian cancer. Factors that stop ovulation or reduce the number of lifetime ovulations, reduce the risk:
- Combined contraceptive pill
- Breastfeeding
- Pregnancy

Presentation

Ovarian cancer can present with non-specific symptoms. In older women, keep the possibility of ovarian cancer in mind and have a low threshold for considering further investigations. Symptoms that may indicate ovarian cancer include:
- Abdominal bloating
- Early satiety (feeling full after eating)
- Loss of appetite
- Pelvic pain
- Urinary symptoms (frequency / urgency)
- Weight loss
- Abdominal or pelvic mass
- Ascites

An ovarian mass may press on the **obturator nerve** and cause referred **hip** or **groin pain**. The obturator nerve passes along the inside of the pelvic, lateral to the ovaries, where an ovarian mass can compress it.

Referral Criteria

The NICE "*suspected cancer: recognition and referral*" guidelines (2015) outlines the key referral criteria and red flags for ovarian cancer. They recommend either referring directly on a 2-week-wait urgent cancer referral or carrying out initial investigations in primary care depending on the presentation.

Refer directly on a **2-week-wait** referral if a physical examination reveals:
- Ascites
- Pelvic mass (unless clearly due to fibroids)
- Abdominal mass

Carry out further investigations before referral in women presenting with symptoms of possible ovarian cancer, starting with a CA125 blood test. This is particularly important in women over 50 years presenting with:
- New symptoms of IBS / change in bowel habit
- Abdominal bloating
- Early satiety
- Pelvic pain
- Urinary frequency or urgency
- Weight loss

Investigations

The initial investigations in primary or secondary care are:
- CA125 blood test (>35 IU/mL is significant)
- Pelvic ultrasound

The **risk of malignancy index** (**RMI**) estimates the risk of an ovarian mass being malignant, taking account of three things:
- Menopausal status
- Ultrasound findings
- CA125 level

Further investigations in secondary care include:
- **CT scan** to establish the diagnosis and stage the cancer
- **Histology** (tissue sample) using a CT guided biopsy, laparoscopy or laparotomy
- **Paracentesis** (ascitic tap) can be used to test the ascitic fluid for cancer cells

Women under 40 years with a **complex ovarian mass** require tumour markers for a possible **germ cell tumour**:
- **Alpha-fetoprotein (α-FP)**
- **Human chorionic gonadotropin (HCG)**

Causes of Raised CA125

CA125 is a tumour marker for **epithelial cell** ovarian cancer. It is not very specific, and there are many non-malignant causes of a raised CA125:
- Endometriosis
- Fibroids
- Adenomyosis
- Pelvic infection
- Liver disease
- Pregnancy

Staging

The **International Federation of Gynaecology and Obstetrics** (**FIGO**) staging system is used to stage ovarian cancer. A very simplified version of this staging system is:
- Stage 1: Confined to the ovary
- Stage 2: Spread past the ovary but inside the pelvis
- Stage 3: Spread past the pelvis but inside the abdomen
- Stage 4: Spread outside the abdomen (distant metastasis)

Management

Ovarian cancer will be managed by a specialist **gynaecology oncology MDT**. It usually involves a combination of **surgery** and **chemotherapy**.

Vulval Cancer

Vulval cancer is rare compared with other gynaecological cancers. Around 90% are **squamous cell carcinomas**. Less commonly, they can be **malignant melanomas**.

Risk Factors

- Advanced age (particularly over 75 years)
- Immunosuppression
- Human papillomavirus (HPV) infection
- **Lichen sclerosus**

Around 5% of women with **lichen sclerosus** get vulval cancer.

Vulval Intraepithelial Neoplasia

Vulval intraepithelial neoplasia (**VIN**) is a premalignant condition affecting the **squamous epithelium** of the skin that can precede vulval cancer. VIN is similar to the premalignant condition that comes before cervical cancer (cervical intraepithelial neoplasia).

High grade squamous intraepithelial lesion is a type of VIN associated with HPV infection that typically occurs in younger women aged 35 - 50 years.

Differentiated VIN is an alternative type of VIN associated with lichen sclerosus and typically occurs in women aged 50 - 60 years.

A biopsy is required to diagnose VIN. A specialist will coordinate management. Treatment options include:
- **Watch and wait** with close followup
- **Wide local excision** (surgery) to remove the lesion
- **Imiquimod** cream
- **Laser ablation**

Presentation

Vulval cancer may be an incidental finding in older women, for example, during catheterisation in a patient with dementia.

Vulval cancer may present with symptoms of:
- Vulval lump
- Ulceration
- Bleeding
- Pain
- Itching
- Lymphadenopathy in the groin

Vulval cancer most frequently affects the **labia majora**, giving an appearance of:
- Irregular mass
- Fungating lesion
- Ulceration
- Bleeding

Management

Suspected vulval cancer should be referred on a **2-week-wait** urgent cancer referral.

Establishing the diagnosis and staging involves:
- **Biopsy** of the lesion
- **Sentinel node biopsy** to demonstrate lymph node spread
- Further imaging for staging (e.g. CT abdomen and pelvis)

The **International Federation of Gynaecology and Obstetrics** (**FIGO**) system is used to stage vulval cancer.

Management depends on the stage, and may involve:
- Wide local excision to remove the cancer
- Groin lymph node dissection
- Chemotherapy
- Radiotherapy

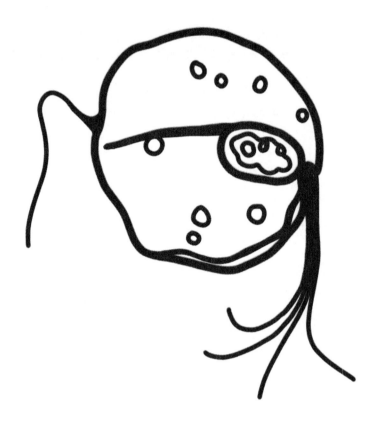

GENITOURINARY MEDICINE

4.1	Bacterial Vaginosis	83
4.2	Candidiasis	84
4.3	Chlamydia	86
4.4	Gonorrhoea	89
4.5	Mycoplasma Genitalium	91
4.6	Pelvic Inflammatory Disease	92
4.7	Trichomoniasis	94
4.8	Genital Herpes	95
4.9	HIV	97
4.10	Syphilis	100

Bacterial Vaginosis

Bacterial vaginosis (**BV**) refers to an overgrowth of bacteria in the vagina, specifically **anaerobic bacteria**. It is not a sexually transmitted infection. It is caused by a **loss** of the **lactobacilli** "friendly bacteria" in the vagina. Bacterial vaginosis can increase the risk of women developing sexually transmitted infections.

Lactobacilli are the main component of the healthy vaginal **bacterial flora**. These bacteria produce **lactic acid** that keeps the **vaginal pH** low (under 4.5). The acidic environment prevents other bacteria from overgrowing. When there are reduced numbers of lactobacilli in the vagina, the **pH rises**. This more **alkaline** environment enables **anaerobic bacteria** to multiply.

Examples of anaerobic bacteria associated with bacterial vaginosis are:
- **Gardnerella vaginalis** (most common)
- **Mycoplasma hominis**
- **Prevotella** species

It is worth remembering that bacterial vaginosis can occur alongside other infections, including candidiasis, chlamydia and gonorrhoea.

Risk Factors

There are a number of factors that increase the risk of developing bacterial vaginosis:
- Multiple sexual partners (although it is not sexually transmitted)
- Excessive vaginal cleaning (douching, use of cleaning products and vaginal washes)
- Recent antibiotics
- Smoking
- Copper coil

Bacterial vaginosis occurs less frequently in women taking the combined pill or using condoms effectively.

TOM TIP: When taking a history from someone with typical symptoms of bacterial vaginosis, the diagnosis can be quite obvious based on the fishy-smelling discharge. The thing that scores you points in your exams and is critical in practice is to assess for causes and give advice. For example, sensitively ask about the use of soaps to clean the vagina and vaginal douching and provide information about how these can increase the risk.

Presentation

The standard presenting feature of bacterial vaginosis is a **fishy-smelling** watery grey or white vaginal discharge. Half of women with BV are asymptomatic.

Itching, irritation and pain are not typically associated with BV and suggest an alternative cause or co-occurring infection.

A **speculum examination** can be performed to confirm the typical discharge, complete a high vaginal swab and exclude other causes of symptoms. Examination is not always required where the symptoms are typical, and the women is low risk for sexually transmitted infections.

Investigations

Vaginal pH can be tested using a swab and pH paper. The normal vaginal pH is 3.5 - 4.5. BV occurs with a pH above 4.5.

A standard charcoal *vaginal swab* can be taken for *microscopy*. This can be a *high vaginal swab* taken during a speculum examination or a *self-taken low vaginal swab*.

Bacterial vaginosis gives "*clue cells*" on microscopy. Clue cells are epithelial cells from the cervix that have bacteria stuck inside them, usually *Gardnerella vaginalis*.

TOM TIP: Remember that clue cells on microscopy indicate bacterial vaginosis. This is a common association tested in MCQ exams.

Management

Asymptomatic BV does not usually require treatment. Additionally, it may resolve without treatment.

Metronidazole is the antibiotic of choice for treating bacterial vaginosis. Metronidazole specifically targets anaerobic bacteria. It is given *orally*, or by *vaginal gel*. *Clindamycin* is an alternative but less optimal antibiotic choice.

Always assess the risk of additional pelvic infections, with swabs for *chlamydia* and *gonorrhoea* where appropriate.

Provide advice and information about measures that can reduce the risk of further episodes of bacterial vaginosis, such as avoiding vaginal irrigation or cleaning with soaps that may disrupt the natural flora.

TOM TIP: Whenever prescribing metronidazole advise patients to avoid alcohol for the duration of treatment. This is a crucial association you should remember, and something examiners will look out for when you are explaining the treatment to a patient. Alcohol and metronidazole can cause a "disulfiram-like reaction", with nausea and vomiting, flushing and sometimes severe symptoms of shock and angioedema.

Complications

Bacterial vaginosis can increase the risk of catching *sexually transmitted infections*, including *chlamydia*, *gonorrhoea* and *HIV*.

It is also associated with several complications in pregnant women:
- Miscarriage
- Preterm delivery
- Premature rupture of membranes
- Chorioamnionitis
- Low birth weight
- Postpartum endometritis

Candidiasis

Vaginal candidiasis is commonly referred to as "thrush". It refers to vaginal infection with a yeast of the *Candida* family. The most common is *Candida albicans*.

Candida may *colonise* the vagina without causing symptoms. It then progresses to infection when the right environment occurs, for example, during pregnancy or after treatment with broad-spectrum antibiotics that alter the vaginal flora.

Risk Factors

- Pregnancy
- Poorly controlled diabetes
- Immunosuppression (e.g. using corticosteroids)
- Broad-spectrum antibiotics

Presentation

The symptoms of vaginal candidiasis are:
- Thick, white discharge that does not typically smell
- Vulval and vaginal itching, irritation or discomfort

More severe infection can lead to:
- Erythema
- Fissures
- Oedema
- Pain during sex (dyspareunia)
- Dysuria
- Excoriation

Investigations

Often treatment for candidiasis is started empirically, based on the presentation.

Testing the **vaginal pH** using a swab and pH paper can be helpful in differentiating between **bacterial vaginosis** and **trichomonas** (pH > 4.5), and **candidiasis** (pH < 4.5).

A *charcoal swab* with *microscopy* can confirm the diagnosis.

Management Options

Treatment of candidiasis is with antifungal medications. These can be delivered in several ways:
- **Antifungal cream** (i.e. clotrimazole) inserted into the vagina with an applicator
- **Antifungal pessary** (i.e. clotrimazole)
- **Oral antifungal tablets** (i.e. fluconazole)

The **NICE Clinical Knowledge Summaries** (2017) recommend for initial uncomplicated cases the options of:
- A single dose of intravaginal clotrimazole cream (5g of 10% cream) at night
- A single dose of clotrimazole pessary (500mg) at night
- Three doses of clotrimazole pessaries (200mg) over three nights
- A single dose of oral fluconazole (150mg)

Canesten Duo is a standard **over-the-counter** treatment worth knowing. It contains a single fluconazole tablet and clotrimazole cream to use externally for vulval symptoms.

They also recommend **recurrent infections** (more than 4 in a year) can be treated with an induction and maintenance regime over six months with oral or vaginal antifungal medications. This is an off-label use.

Warn women that antifungal creams and pessaries can damage latex condoms and prevent spermicides from working, so alternative contraceptive is required for at least five days after use.

Chlamydia

Chlamydia trachomatis is a **gram-negative** bacteria. It is an **intracellular organism**, meaning it enters and replicates within cells before rupturing the cell and spreading to others. Chlamydia is the most common sexually transmitted infection in the UK and a significant cause of infertility.

Being young, sexually active and having multiple partners increase the risk of catching the infection. A large number of cases are asymptomatic (50% in men and 75% in woman). Asymptomatic patients can still pass the infection on.

National Chlamydia Screening Programm

Public Health England has set out a **National Chlamydia Screening Programme** (**NCSP**). This program aims to screen every sexually active person under 25 years of age for chlamydia **annually** or when they change their sexual partner. Everyone that tests positive should have a re-test three months after treatment. This re-testing is to ensure they have not contracted chlamydia again, rather than to check the treatment has worked.

In general, when a patient attends a GUM clinic for STI screening, as a minimum, they are tested for:
- Chlamydia
- Gonorrhoea
- Syphilis (blood test)
- HIV (blood test)

Swabs

It can be tricky to get your head around the swabs used for sexual health screening. There are many different swab types and uses. The FSRH clinical guideline on vaginal discharge (2012) has helpful guidance on the investigation with different swabs in different clinical scenarios. There are two types of swabs involved in sexual health testing:
- **Charcoal swabs**
- **Nucleic acid amplification test** (**NAAT**) swabs

Charcoal swabs allow for **microscopy** (looking at the sample under the microscope), **culture** (growing the organism) and **sensitivities** (testing which antibiotics are effective against the bacteria). Charcoal swabs look like a long cotton bud that goes into a tube with a black transport medium at the end. The transport medium is called **Amies transport medium**, and contains a chemical solution for keeping microorganisms alive during transport.

Microscopy involves **gram staining** and examination under a microscope. A stain is used to highlight different types of bacteria with different colours. Charcoal swabs can be used for **endocervical swabs** and **high vaginal swabs** (**HVS**). Charcoal swabs can confirm:
- Bacterial vaginosis
- Candidiasis
- **Gonorrhoea** (specifically on an endocervical swab)
- **Trichomonas vaginalis** (specifically a swab from the posterior fornix)
- Other bacteria, such as **group B streptococcus** (**GBS**)

Nucleic acid amplification tests (**NAAT**) check directly for the **DNA** or **RNA** of the organism. NAAT testing is used to test specifically for **chlamydia** and **gonorrhoea**. They are not useful for other pelvic infections. In women, a NAAT test can be performed on a **vulvovaginal swab** (a self-taken lower vaginal swab), an **endocervical swab** or a **first-catch urine** sample. The order of preference is endocervical, vulvovaginal, and then urine. In men, a NAAT test can be performed on a **first-catch urine** sample or a **urethral swab**. It is worth noting that the NAAT swabs will specify on the packet whether the swabs are for endocervical, vulvovaginal or urethral use. A specific kit is used for first-catch urine NATT testing.

Rectal and **pharyngeal** NAAT swabs can also be taken to diagnose **chlamydia** in the **rectum** and **throat**. Consider these swabs where **anal** or **oral** sex has occurred.

Where **gonorrhoea** is suspected or demonstrated on a NAAT test, an **endocervical charcoal swab** is required for **microscopy**, **culture** and **sensitivities**.

Presentation

The majority of cases of chlamydia in women are asymptomatic. Consider chlamydia in women that are sexually active and present with:
- Abnormal vaginal discharge
- Pelvic pain
- Abnormal vaginal bleeding (intermenstrual or postcoital)
- Painful sex (dyspareunia)
- Painful urination (dysuria)

Consider chlamydia in men that are sexually active and present with:
- Urethral discharge or discomfort
- Painful urination (dysuria)
- Epididymo-orchitis
- Reactive arthritis

It is worth considering **rectal chlamydia** and **lymphogranuloma venereum** in patients presenting with anorectal symptoms, such as discomfort, discharge, bleeding or a change in bowel habits.

Examination Findings

- Pelvic or abdominal tenderness
- Cervical motion tenderness (cervical excitation)
- Inflamed cervix (cervicitis)
- Purulent discharge

Diagnosis

Nucleic acid amplification tests (NAAT) are used to diagnose chlamydia. This can involve a:
- Vulvovaginal swab
- Endocervical swab
- First-catch urine sample (in women or men)
- Urethral swab in men
- Rectal swab (after anal sex)
- Pharyngeal swab (after oral sex)

Management

This section is based on the **British Association for Sexual Health and HIV** (**BASHH**) guidelines (published 2015, updated 2018). Always check local and national guidelines before treating patients. This is a summary to help with your learning and exam preparation.

First-line for uncomplicated chlamydia infection is **doxycycline 100mg twice a day for 7 days**.

The guidelines previously recommended a single dose of azithromycin 1g orally as an alternative. This recommendation has been removed due to **Mycoplasma genitalium** resistance to azithromycin, and azithromycin being less effective for rectal chlamydia infection.

Doxycycline is contraindicated in pregnancy and breastfeeding. Alternatives options listed in the BASHH guidelines (always check guidelines) for treatment in pregnant or breastfeeding women are:
- Azithromycin 1g stat then 500mg once a day for 2 days
- Erythromycin 500mg four times daily for 7 days
- Erythromycin 500mg twice daily for 14 days
- Amoxicillin 500mg three times daily for 7 days

A **test of cure** is not routinely recommended. However, a test of cure should be used for rectal cases of chlamydia, in pregnancy and where symptoms persist.

Other factors to consider are:
- Abstain from sex for seven days of treatment of all partners to reduce the risk of re-infection
- Refer all patients to **genitourinary medicine** (**GUM**) for contact tracing and notification of sexual partners
- Test for and treat any other sexually transmitted infections
- Provide advice about ways to prevent future infection
- Consider safeguarding issues and sexual abuse in children and young people

Complications

There are a large number of complications from infection with chlamydia:
- Pelvic inflammatory disease
- Chronic pelvic pain
- Infertility
- Ectopic pregnancy
- Epididymo-orchitis
- Conjunctivitis
- Lymphogranuloma venereum
- Reactive arthritis

Pregnancy-related complications include:
- Preterm delivery
- Premature rupture of membranes
- Low birth weight
- Postpartum endometritis
- Neonatal infection (conjunctivitis and pneumonia)

Lymphogranuloma Venereum

Lymphogranuloma venereum (**LGV**) is a condition affecting the lymphoid tissue around the site of infection with chlamydia. It most commonly occurs in men who have sex with men (MSM). LGV occurs in three stages:

The **primary stage** involves a **painless ulcer** (**primary lesion**). This typically occurs on the penis in men, vaginal wall in women or rectum after anal sex.

The **secondary stage** involves **lymphadenitis**. This is swelling, inflammation and pain in the lymph nodes infected with the bacteria. The inguinal or femoral lymph nodes may be affected.

The **tertiary stage** involves inflammation of the rectum (**proctitis**) and anus. **Proctocolitis** leads to anal pain, change in bowel habit, **tenesmus** and discharge. Tenesmus is a feeling of needing to empty the bowels, even after completing a bowel motion.

Doxycycline 100mg twice daily for 21 days is the first-line treatment for LGV recommended by BASHH. Erythromycin, azithromycin and ofloxacin are alternatives.

Chlamydial Conjunctivitis

Chlamydia can infect the conjunctiva of the eye. Conjunctival infection is usually a result of sexual activity, when genital fluid comes in contact with the eye, for example, through hand-to-eye spread. It presents with chronic erythema, irritation and discharge lasting more than two weeks. Most cases are unilateral.

Chlamydial conjunctivitis occurs more frequently in young adults. It can also affect neonates with mothers infected with chlamydia. Gonococcal conjunctivitis is a crucial differential diagnosis and should be tested.

Gonorrhoea

Neisseria gonorrhoeae is a **Gram-negative diplococcus** bacteria. It infects **mucous membranes** with a **columnar epithelium**, such as the **endocervix** in women, **urethra**, **rectum**, **conjunctiva** and **pharynx**. It spreads via contact with mucous secretions from infected areas.

Gonorrhoea is a **sexually transmitted infection**. Being young, sexually active and having multiple partners increases the risk of infection with gonorrhoea. Having other sexually transmitted infections, such as chlamydia or HIV, also increases the risk.

There is a high level of **antibiotic resistance** with gonorrhoea. Traditionally **ciprofloxacin** or **azithromycin** were used to treat gonorrhoea. However, there are now high levels of resistance to these antibiotics.

Presentation

Infection with gonorrhoea is more likely to be symptomatic than infection with chlamydia. 90% of men and 50% of women are symptomatic. The presentation will vary depending on the site. Female genital infections can present with:
- Odourless purulent discharge, possibly green or yellow
- Dysuria
- Pelvic pain

Male genital infections can present with:
- Odourless purulent discharge, possibly green or yellow
- Dysuria
- Testicular pain or swelling (**epididymo-orchitis**)

Rectal infection may cause anal or rectal discomfort and discharge, but is often asymptomatic. **Pharyngeal infection** may cause a sore throat, but is often asymptomatic. **Prostatitis** causes perineal pain, urinary symptoms and prostate tenderness on examination. **Conjunctivitis** causes erythema and a purulent discharge.

Diagnosis

Nucleic acid amplification testing (**NATT**) is use to detect the **RNA** or **DNA** of gonorrhoea. Genital infection can be diagnosed with **endocervical**, **vulvovaginal** or **urethral** swabs, or in a **first-catch urine** sample. **Rectal** and **pharyngeal** swab are recommended in all **men who have sex with men** (**MSM**), and in those with risk factors (e.g. anal and oral sex) or symptoms of infection in these areas.

A standard charcoal **endocervical swab** should be taken for **microscopy**, **culture** and **antibiotic sensitivities** before initiating antibiotics. This is particularly important given the high rates of antibiotic resistance.

TOM TIP: It is worth remembering that NATT tests are used to check if a gonococcal infection is present or not by looking for gonococcal RNA or DNA. They do not provide any information about the specific bacteria and their antibiotic sensitivities and resistance. This is why a standard charcoal swab for microscopy, culture and sensitivities is so essential, to guide the choice of antibiotics to use in treatment.

Management

This section is based on the **British Association for Sexual Health and HIV** (**BASHH**) guidelines (2018). Given local differences in antibiotic resistances and frequently changing regimes, always look up the latest local and national guidelines when treating patients. This is a summary to help with your learning and exam preparation.

Patients should be referred to GUM clinics (or local equivalent) to **coordinate testing**, **treatment** and **contact tracing**. Management depends on whether antibiotic sensitivities are known. For uncomplicated gonococcal infections:
- A single dose of **intramuscular ceftriaxone** 1g if the sensitivities are NOT known
- A single dose of **oral ciprofloxacin** 500mg if the sensitivities ARE known

Different regimes are recommended for complicated infections, infections in other sites and pregnant women. Most regimes involve a single dose of intramuscular ceftriaxone.

All patients should have a follow up "**test of cure**" given the high antibiotic resistance. This is with NAAT testing if they are asymptomatic, or cultures where they are symptomatic. BASHH recommend a test of cure **at least**:
- 72 hours after treatment for culture
- 7 days after treatment for RNA NATT
- 14 days after treatment for DNA NATT

Other factors to consider are:
- Abstain from sex for seven days of treatment of all partners to reduce the risk of re-infection
- Test for and treat any other sexually transmitted infections
- Provide advice about ways to prevent future infection
- Consider safeguarding issues and sexual abuse in children and young people

Complications

- Pelvic inflammatory disease
- Chronic pelvic pain
- Infertility
- Epididymo-orchitis (men)
- Prostatitis (men)
- Conjunctivitis
- Urethral strictures
- Disseminated gonococcal infection
- Skin lesions
- Fitz-Hugh-Curtis syndrome
- Septic arthritis
- Endocarditis

A key complication to remember is **gonococcal conjunctivitis** in a neonate. Gonococcal infection is contracted from the mother during birth. Neonatal conjunctivitis is called **ophthalmia neonatorum**. This is a medical emergency and is associated with sepsis, perforation of the eye and blindness.

Disseminated Gonococcal Infection

Disseminated gonococcal infection (**GDI**) is a complication of untreated gonococcal infection, where the bacteria spreads to the skin and joints. It causes:
- Various non-specific **skin lesions**
- **Polyarthralgia** (joint aches and pains)
- **Migratory polyarthritis** (arthritis that moves)
- **Tenosynovitis**
- **Systemic symptoms** such as fever and fatigue

Mycoplasma Genitalium

Mycoplasma genitalium (**MG**) is a bacteria that causes **non-gonococcal urethritis**. It is a **sexually transmitted infection**. There are developing problems with antibiotic resistance, particularly with azithromycin.

Most cases of MG do not cause symptoms. The presentation is very similar to chlamydia, and patients may be infected with both organisms. **Urethritis** is a key feature.

Mycoplasma genitalium infection may lead to:
- Urethritis
- Epididymitis
- Cervicitis
- Endometritis
- Pelvic inflammatory disease
- Reactive arthritis
- Preterm delivery in pregnancy
- Tubal infertility

Investigations

Traditional cultures are not helpful in isolating MG, as it is a very slow-growing organism. Therefore, testing involves **nucleic acid amplification tests** (**NAAT**) to look specifically for the DNA or RNA if the bacteria.

The samples recommended by **BASHH guidelines** (2018) are:
- **First urine sample** in the morning for men
- **Vaginal swabs** (can be self-taken) for women

The guideline recommends checking every positive sample for **macrolide resistance**, and performing a "**test of cure**" after treatment in every positive patient.

Management

The **BASHH guidelines** (2018) recommend a course of **doxycycline** followed by **azithromycin** for uncomplicated genital infections:
- **Doxycycline** 100mg twice daily for 7 days then;
- **Azithromycin** 1g stat then 500mg once a day for 2 days (unless it is known to be resistant to macrolides)

Moxifloxacin is used as an alternative or in complicated infections. Azithromycin alone is used in pregnancy and breastfeeding (remember doxycycline is contraindicated).

Pelvic Inflammatory Disease

Pelvic inflammatory disease (**PID**) is inflammation and infection of the organs of the pelvis, caused by infection spreading up through the cervix. It is a significant cause of **tubal infertility** and **chronic pelvic pain**.

It is worth remembering the technical terms for the affected organs:
- **Endometritis** is inflammation of the **endometrium**
- **Salpingitis** is inflammation of the **fallopian tubes**
- **Oophoritis** is inflammation of the **ovaries**
- **Parametritis** is inflammation of the **parametrium**, which is the **connective tissue** around the uterus
- **Peritonitis** is inflammation of the **peritoneal membrane**

Causes

Most cases of pelvic inflammatory disease are caused by one of the sexually transmitted pelvic infections:
- **Neisseria gonorrhoeae** tends to produce more severe PID
- **Chlamydia trachomatis**
- **Mycoplasma genitalium**

Pelvic inflammatory disease can less commonly be caused by non-sexually transmitted infections, such as:
- **Gardnerella vaginalis** (associated with **bacterial vaginosis**)
- **Haemophilus influenzae** (a bacteria often associated with respiratory infections)
- **Escherichia coli** (an enteric bacteria commonly associated with urinary tract infections)

Risk Factors

The risk factors for pelvic inflammatory disease are the same as any other sexually transmitted infection:
- Not using barrier contraception
- Multiple sexual partners
- Younger age
- Existing sexually transmitted infections
- Previous pelvic inflammatory disease
- Intrauterine device (e.g. copper coil)

Presentation

Women may present with symptoms of:
- Pelvic or lower abdominal pain
- Abnormal vaginal discharge
- Abnormal bleeding (intermenstrual or postcoital)
- Pain during sex (dyspareunia)
- Fever
- Dysuria

Examination findings may reveal:
- Pelvic tenderness
- Cervical motion tenderness (cervical excitation)
- Inflamed cervix (cervicitis)
- Purulent discharge

Patients may have a fever and other signs of sepsis.

Investigations

Patients with pelvic inflammatory disease should have testing for causative organisms and other sexually transmitted infections:
- NAAT swabs for gonorrhoea and chlamydia
- NAAT swabs for Mycoplasma genitalium if available
- HIV test
- Syphilis test

A **high vaginal swab** can be used to look for **bacterial vaginosis**, **candidiasis** and **trichomoniasis**.

A microscope can be used to look for **pus cells** on swabs from the vagina or endocervix. The absence of pus cells is useful for excluding PID.

A **pregnancy test** should be performed on sexually active women presenting with lower abdominal pain to exclude an **ectopic pregnancy**.

Inflammatory markers (CRP and ESR) are raised in PID and can help support the diagnosis.

Management

Where appropriate patients should be referred to a **genitourinary medicine** (**GUM**) specialist service for management and **contact tracing**. Antibiotics are started empirically, before swab results are obtained, to avoid delay and complications.

Antibiotics will depend on local and national guidelines. The **BASSH guidelines** (published 2018, updated 2019) suggest various inpatient and outpatient regimes to cover possible causative organisms. One suggested outpatient regime (listed here to help your understanding and not as a guide to treatment) is:
- A single dose of **intramuscular ceftriaxone** 1g (to cover **gonorrhoea**)
- **Doxycycline** 100mg twice daily for 14 days (to cover **chlamydia** and **Mycoplasma genitalium**)
- **Metronidazole** 400mg twice daily for 14 days (to cover **anaerobes** such as **Gardnerella vaginalis**)

Ceftriaxone and doxycycline will cover many other bacteria, including **H. influenzae** and **E. coli**.

More severe cases, particularly where there are signs of sepsis or the patient is pregnant, require admission to hospital for IV antibiotics. Where a pelvic abscess develops, this may need drainage by interventional radiology or surgery.

Complications

- Sepsis
- Abscess
- Infertility
- Chronic pelvic pain
- Ectopic pregnancy
- Fitz-Hugh-Curtis syndrome

Fitz-Hugh-Curtis Syndrome

Fitz-Hugh-Curtis syndrome is a complication of pelvic inflammatory disease. It is caused by inflammation and infection of the **liver capsule** (**Glisson's capsule**), leading to adhesions between the liver and peritoneum. Bacteria may spread from the pelvis via the peritoneal cavity, lymphatic system or blood.

Fitz-Hugh-Curtis syndrome results in **right upper quadrant pain** that can be referred to the right shoulder tip if there is diaphragmatic irritation. **Laparoscopy** can be used to visualise and also treat the adhesions by **adhesiolysis**.

Trichomoniasis

Trichomonas vaginalis is a type of parasite spread through sexual intercourse. Trichomonas is classed as a **protozoan**, and is a single-celled organism with **flagella**. Flagella are appendages stretching from the body, similar to limbs. Trichomonas has four flagella at the front and a single flagellum at the back, giving a characteristic appearance to the organism. The flagella are used for movement, attaching to tissues and causing damage.

Trichomonas is spread through sexual activity. It lives in the urethra of men and women, and the vagina of women.

Trichomonas can increase the risk of:
- **Contracting HIV** by damaging the vaginal mucosa
- **Bacterial vaginosis**
- **Cervical cancer**
- **Pelvic inflammatory disease**
- **Pregnancy-related complications**, such as preterm delivery

Presentation

Up to 50% of cases of trichomoniasis are asymptomatic. When symptoms occur, they are non-specific:
- Vaginal discharge
- Itching
- Dysuria (painful urination)
- Dyspareunia (painful sex)
- Balanitis (inflammation to the glans penis)

The typical description of the vaginal discharge is **frothy** and **yellow-green**, although this can vary significantly. It may have a **fishy smell**.

Examination of the cervix can reveal a characteristic "**strawberry cervix**" (also called **colpitis macularis**). A strawberry cervix is caused by inflammation (cervicitis) relating to the trichomonas infection. There are tiny haemorrhages across the surface of the cervix, giving the appearance of a strawberry.

Testing the **vaginal pH** will reveal a raised ph (above 4.5), similar to bacterial vaginosis.

Diagnosis

The diagnosis can be confirmed with a standard **charcoal swab** with **microscopy** (examination under a microscope).

Swabs should be taken from the **posterior fornix of the vagina** (behind the cervix) in women. A **self-taken low vaginal swab** may be used as an alternative.

A **urethral swab** or **first-catch urine** is used in men.

Management

Patients should be referred to a **genitourinary medicine** (**GUM**) specialist service for diagnosis, treatment and **contact tracing**.

Treatment is with **metronidazole**.

Genital Herpes

The **herpes simplex virus** (**HSV**) is commonly responsible for both **cold sores** (**herpes labialis**) and **genital herpes**. There are two main strains, **HSV-1** and **HSV-2**. Both strains are common in the UK, and many people are infected without experiencing any symptoms. After an initial infection, the virus becomes **latent** in the associated **sensory nerve ganglia**. Typically this is the **trigeminal nerve ganglion** with cold sores, and the **sacral nerve ganglia** with genital herpes.

The herpes simplex virus can also cause **aphthous ulcers** (small painful oral sores in the mouth), **herpes keratitis** (inflammation of the cornea in the eye) and **herpetic whitlow** (a painful skin lesion on a finger or thumb).

The herpes simplex virus is spread through direct contact with affected **mucous membranes**, or **viral shedding** in **mucous secretions**. The virus can be shed even when no symptoms are present, meaning it can be contracted from asymptomatic individuals. Asymptomatic shedding is more common in the first 12 months of infection, and where recurrent symptoms are present.

HSV-1 is most associated with **cold sores**. It is often contracted initially in childhood (before five years), remains dormant in the **trigeminal nerve ganglion** and reactivates as cold sores, particularly in times of stress. **Genital herpes** caused by HSV-1 is usually contracted through **oro-genital sex**, where the virus spreads from a person with an oral infection to the person that develops the genital infection.

HSV-2 typically causes **genital herpes** and is mostly a **sexually transmitted infection**. It can also cause lesions in the mouth.

Presentation of Genital Herpes

Patients affected by herpes simplex may display no symptoms, or develop symptoms months or years after an initial infection when the latent virus is reactivated.

The symptoms of an initial infection with genital herpes usually appear within two weeks. The initial episode is often the most severe, and recurrent episodes are more mild.

Signs and symptoms include:
- **Ulcers** or **blistering lesions** affecting the genital area
- **Neuropathic** type pain (tingling, burning or shooting)
- **Flu-like** symptoms (e.g. fatigue and headaches)
- **Dysuria** (painful urination)
- **Inguinal lymphadenopathy**

Symptoms can last three weeks in a primary infection. Recurrent episodes are usually milder and resolve more quickly.

Diagnosis

Ask about sexual contacts, including those with cold sores, to establish a possible source of transmission. They may have caught the infection from someone unaware they are infected and not experiencing any symptoms.

The diagnosis can be made **clinically** based on the history and examination findings.

A **viral PCR** swab from a lesion can confirm the diagnosis and causative organism.

Management

Patients should be referred to a **genitourinary medicine** (**GUM**) specialist service.

Aciclovir is used to treat genital herpes. There are various aciclovir regimes listed in the BNF, depending on the individual circumstances. Alternatives are valaciclovir and famciclovir.

Additional measures, including to manage the symptoms include:
- Paracetamol
- Topical lidocaine 2% gel (e.g. **Instillagel**)
- Cleaning with warm salt water
- Topical vaseline
- Additional oral fluids
- Wear loose clothing
- Avoid intercourse with symptoms

Pregnancy and Genital Herpes

Genital herpes is **not** known to cause pregnancy-related complications or congenital abnormalities. The main issue with genital herpes during pregnancy is the risk of **neonatal herpes simplex infection** contracted during labour and delivery. Neonatal herpes simplex infection has high **morbidity** and **mortality**. Neonatal infection should be avoided as much as possible and treated early if identified.

After an initial infection with genital herpes, the woman will develop **antibodies** to the virus. During pregnancy, these **antibodies** can cross the **placenta** into the fetus. This gives the fetus **passive immunity** to the virus, and protects the baby during labour and delivery.

Management of genital herpes in pregnancy depends on whether it is the first episode of genital herpes (**primary infection**) or **recurrent genital herpes**. There are guidelines on genital herpes from the **RCOG** (2014). Always check local and national guidelines when treating patients. **Aciclovir** is not known to be harmful in pregnancy.

Primary genital herpes contracted **before 28 weeks gestation** is treated with **aciclovir** during the initial infection. This is followed by regular **prophylactic aciclovir** starting from 36 weeks gestation onwards to reduce the risk of genital lesions during labour and delivery. Women that are asymptomatic at delivery can have a vaginal delivery (provided it is more than six weeks after the initial infection). Caesarean section is recommended when symptoms are present.

Primary genital herpes contracted **after 28 weeks gestation** is treated with aciclovir during the initial infection followed immediately by regular **prophylactic aciclovir**. **Caesarean section** is recommended in all cases to reduce the risk of neonatal infection.

Recurrent genital herpes in pregnancy, where the woman is known to have genital herpes before the pregnancy, carries a low risk of neonatal infection (0-3%), even if the lesions are present during delivery. Regular **prophylactic aciclovir** is considered from 36 weeks gestation to reduce the risk of symptoms at the time of delivery.

HIV

HIV refers to the **human immunodeficiency virus**. Being infected with HIV is referred to as being **HIV positive**.

AIDS refers to **acquired immunodeficiency syndrome**. AIDS occurs as a HIV infection progresses, and the person becomes **immunodeficient**. This immunodeficiency leads to opportunistic infections and several **AIDS-defining illnesses**, such as **Kaposi's sarcoma**. AIDS is now mostly referred to as **late-stage HIV**.

Basics

HIV is an **RNA retrovirus**. **HIV-1** is the most common type, and **HIV-2** is rare outside West Africa. The virus enters and destroys the **CD4 T-helper cells** of the immune system.

An initial **seroconversion** flu-like illness occurs within a few weeks of infection. The infection is then asymptomatic until the condition progresses to immunodeficiency. Immunodeficient patients develop **AIDS-defining illnesses** and opportunistic infections. This progression occurs potentially years after the initial infection.

Transmission

HIV is not transmitted through day-to-day activities, including kissing. It is spread through:
- Unprotected anal, vaginal or oral sexual activity
- Mother to child at any stage of pregnancy, birth or breastfeeding (called **vertical transmission**)
- Mucous membrane, blood or open wound exposure to infected **blood** or **bodily fluids**, for example, through sharing needles, needle-stick injuries or blood splashed in an eye

AIDS-Defining Illnesses

There is a long list of **AIDS-defining illnesses** associated with **end-stage HIV** infection. These occur where the **CD4 count** has dropped to a level that allows for unusual opportunistic infections and malignancies to appear.

Examples of AIDS-defining illnesses include:
- Kaposi's sarcoma
- Pneumocystis jirovecii pneumonia (PCP)
- Cytomegalovirus infection
- Candidiasis (oesophageal or bronchial)
- Lymphomas
- Tuberculosis

Screening

Many people with HIV do not know they are infected, and these patients are at risk of complications and spreading the disease. Generally, the earlier a patient is diagnosed, the better the outcome. HIV is a treatable condition, and most patients are fit and healthy on treatment.

We should test practically everyone admitted to hospital with an infectious disease for HIV, regardless of their risk factors. Patients with any risk factors should be tested.

It can take up to **three months** to develop antibodies to the virus after infection. Therefore, **HIV antibody tests** can be negative for three months following exposure, and repeat testing is necessary if an initial test is negative within three months of exposure to the virus.

Patients need to give **consent** for a test. **Verbal consent** should be documented before a test. Gaining consent can be as simple as asking "are you happy for us to test you for HIV?" Patients no longer require formal counselling or education before a test.

Testing

Antibody testing is the typical screening test for HIV. This is a simple blood test. Patients can request an antibody testing kit online for **self sampling** at home, which they post to the lab for testing.

Testing for the **p24 antigen** in the blood. This can give a positive result earlier in the infection compared with the antibody test.

PCR testing for the **HIV RNA** levels tests directly for the number of **viral copies** in the blood, giving a **viral load**.

Monitoring

CD4 Count
The CD4 count is the number of CD4 cells in the blood. These are the cells destroyed by the virus. The lower the count, the higher the risk of opportunistic infection:
- 500-1200 cells/mm^3 is the normal range
- Under 200 cells/mm^3 is considered **end-stage HIV** (AIDS) and puts the patient at high risk of opportunistic infections

Viral Load (VL)
Viral load is the number of copies of **HIV RNA** per ml of blood. "**Undetectable**" refers to a viral load below the lab's recordable range (usually 50 – 100 copies/ml). The viral load can be in the hundreds of thousands in untreated HIV.

Treatment

Specialist **HIV**, **infectious disease** or **GUM** centres manage patients with HIV. Treatment involves a combination of **antiretroviral therapy** (**ART**) medications. ART is offered to everyone with a diagnosis of HIV irrespective of **viral load** or **CD4 count**. Some regimes involve only a single combination tablet, taken once daily, with the potential to suppress the infection completely. Specialist blood tests can establish the resistance of each HIV strain to different medications and help tailor treatment. The **BHIVA guidelines** (2015) recommend a starting regime of two **NRTIs** (e.g. tenofovir and emtricitabine) plus a third agent.

Treatment aims to achieve a **normal CD4 count** and **undetectable viral load**. As a general rule, when a patient has a normal CD4 and an undetectable viral load on ART, treat their physical health problems (e.g. routine chest infections) as you would an HIV negative patient. When prescribing for patients on ART, be aware and carefully check for any medication interactions with the HIV therapy.

Highly Active Anti-Retrovirus Therapy (HAART) Medication

There are a number of classes of HAART medications that work slightly differently on the virus:
- Protease inhibitors (PIs)
- Integrase inhibitors (IIs)
- Nucleoside reverse transcriptase inhibitors (NRTIs)
- Non-nucleoside reverse transcriptase inhibitors (NNRTIs)
- Entry inhibitors (EIs)

Additional Management

Prophylactic co-trimoxazole (**Septrin**) is given to patients with a CD4 under 200/mm^3, to protect against **pneumocystis jirovecii pneumonia** (**PCP**).

HIV infection increases the risk of developing **cardiovascular disease**. Patients with HIV have close monitoring of cardiovascular risk factors and blood lipids. Appropriate treatment (e.g. statins) may be required to reduce their risk.

Yearly cervical smears are required for women with HIV. HIV predisposes to developing **human papillomavirus** (**HPV**) infection and **cervical cancer**, so female patients need close monitoring to ensure early detection of these complications.

Vaccinations should be up to date, including influenza, pneumococcal, hepatitis A and B, tetanus, diphtheria and polio vaccines. Patients should avoid **live vaccines**.

Reproductive Health

Advise condoms for vaginal and anal sex, and dams for oral sex, even when both partners are HIV positive. If the viral load is **undetectable**, transmission through unprotected sex is unheard of, even in extensive studies, although infection is not impossible. Partners should have regular HIV tests.

Where the affected partner has an undetectable viral load, unprotected sex and pregnancy may be considered. It is also possible to conceive safely through techniques like **sperm washing** and **IVF**.

Preventing Transmission During Birth

The mother's viral load will determine the mode of delivery:
- **Normal vaginal delivery** is recommended for women with a viral load < 50 copies / ml
- **Caesarean section** is considered in patients with > 50 copies / ml and in all women with > 400 copies / ml
- **IV zidovudine** should be given during the caesarean if the viral load is unknown or there are > 10,000 copies / ml

Prophylaxis treatment may be given to the baby, depending on the mothers viral load:
- Low-risk babies, where the mother's viral load is < 50 copies per ml, are given **zidovudine** for four weeks
- High-risk babies, where the mother's viral load is > 50 copies / ml, are given **zidovudine**, **lamivudine** and **nevirapine** for four weeks

This description of measures to prevent vertical transmission is an over-simplified illustration of the **BHIVA guidelines**. You don't need to know the details for your medical school exams, but it is helpful to be aware of the basic principles.

Breast Feeding

HIV can be transmitted during breastfeeding, even if the mother's viral load is undetectable.

Breastfeeding is not recommended for mothers with HIV. However, if the mother is adamant and the viral load is undetectable, sometimes it is attempted with close monitoring by the HIV team.

Post-Exposure Prophylaxis

Post-exposure prophylaxis (**PEP**) can be used after exposure to HIV to reduce the risk of transmission. PEP is not 100% effective and must be commenced within a short window of opportunity (less than 72 hours). The sooner it is started, the better. A risk assessment of the probability of developing HIV should be balanced against the side effects of PEP.

PEP involves a combination of **ART therapy**. The current regime is **Truvada** (emtricitabine and tenofovir) and **raltegravir** for 28 days.

HIV tests are done **immediately** and also a minimum of **three months** after exposure to confirm a negative status. Individuals should abstain from unprotected sexual activity for a minimum of three months until confirmed as negative.

Syphilis

Syphilis is caused by bacteria called **Treponema pallidum**. This bacteria is a **spirochete**, a type of **spiral-shaped** bacteria. The bacteria gets in through skin or mucous membranes, replicates and then disseminates throughout the body. It is mainly a **sexually transmitted infection**. The incubation period between the initial infection and symptoms is 21 days on average.

Transmission

Syphilis can also be contracted through:
- **Oral**, **vaginal** or **anal sex** involving direct contact with an infected area
- **Vertical transmission** from mother to baby during pregnancy
- **Intravenous drug use**
- **Blood transfusions** and **other transplants** (although this is rare due to screening of blood products)

Stages

Primary syphilis involves a **painless ulcer** called a **chancre** at the original site of infection (usually on the genitals).

Secondary syphilis involves systemic symptoms, particularly of the skin and mucous membranes. These symptoms can resolve after 3 - 12 weeks and the patient can enter the **latent stage**.

Latent syphilis occurs after the secondary stage of syphilis, where symptoms disappear and the patient becomes asymptomatic despite still being infected. **Early latent syphilis** occurs within two years of the initial infection, and **late latent syphilis** occurs from two years after the initial infection onwards.

Tertiary syphilis can occur many years after the initial infection and affect many organs of the body, particularly with the development of **gummas**, and cardiovascular and neurological complications.

Neurosyphilis occurs if the infection involves the **central nervous system**, presenting with neurological symptoms.

Presentation

Primary syphilis can present with:
- A painless genital ulcer (**chancre**). This tends to resolve over 3 - 8 weeks.
- Local lymphadenopathy

Secondary syphilis typically starts after the chancre has healed, with symptoms of:
- Maculopapular rash
- **Condylomata lata** (grey wart-like lesions around the genitals and anus)
- Low-grade fever
- Lymphadenopathy
- Alopecia (localised hair loss)
- Oral lesions

Tertiary syphilis can present with several symptoms depending on the affected organs. Key features to be aware of are:
- **Gummatous lesions** (**gummas** are granulomatous lesions that can affect the skin, organs and bones)
- Aortic aneurysms
- Neurosyphilis

Neurosyphilis can occur at any stage if the infection reaches the central nervous system, and present with symptoms of:
- Headache
- Altered behaviour
- Dementia
- **Tabes dorsalis** (demyelination affecting the spinal cord posterior columns)
- **Ocular syphilis** (affecting the eyes)
- Paralysis
- Sensory impairment

Argyll-Robertson pupil is a specific finding in **neurosyphilis**. It is a **constricted** pupil that **accommodates** when focusing on a near object, but **does not react to light**. They are often irregularly shaped. It is commonly called a "**prostitutes pupil**" due to the relation to neurosyphilis and because "**it accommodates but does not react**".

Diagnosis

Antibody testing for antibodies to the **T. pallidum** bacteria can be used as a screening test for syphilis.

Patients with suspected syphilis or positive antibodies should be referred to a specialist GUM centre for further testing.

Samples from sites of infection can be tested to confirm the presence of **T. pallidum** with:
- **Dark field microscopy**
- **Polymerase chain reaction** (**PCR**)

The **rapid plasma reagin** (**RPR**) and **venereal disease research laboratory** (**VDRL**) tests are two **non-specific** but **sensitive** tests used to assess for active syphilis infection. These tests assess the **quantity of antibodies** being produced by the body to an infection with syphilis. A higher number indicates a greater chance of active disease. These tests involve introducing a sample of serum to a solution containing antigens and assessing the reaction. A more significant reaction suggests a higher quantity of antibodies. The tests are **non-specific**, meaning they often produce **false-positive** results. There is a skill to both performing and interpreting the results of these tests.

Management

All patients should be managed and followed up by a specialist service, such as GUM. As with all sexually transmitted infections, patients need:
- Full screening for other STIs
- Advice about avoiding sexual activity until treated
- Contact tracing
- Prevention of future infections

A single **deep intramuscular** dose of **benzathine benzylpenicillin** (penicillin) is the standard treatment for syphilis.

Alternative regimes and types of penicillin are used in different scenarios, for example, late syphilis and neurosyphilis. Ceftriaxone, amoxicillin and doxycycline are alternatives.

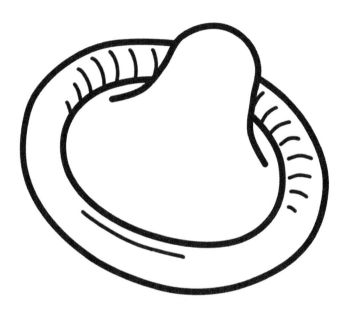

CONTRACEPTION

5.1	Basics of Contraception	104
5.2	Barrier Methods	106
5.3	Combined Oral Contraceptive Pill	107
5.4	Progestogen-Only Pill	111
5.6	Progestogen-Only Injection	113
5.7	Progestogen-Only Implant	115
5.5	Coils	117
5.8	Emergency Contraception	120
5.9	Sterilisation	122
5.10	Consent to Contraception	122

Basics of Contraception

There are many methods of contraception you need to be familiar with. It is a common task in OSCEs to counsel a patient about the different options. This involves discussing:
- Different options
- Suitability (including assessing contraindications and risks)
- Effectiveness
- Mechanism of action
- Instruction on use

It is worth noting that all forms of contraception are available free in the UK on the NHS.

Methods of Contraception

The key contraceptive methods available are:
- Natural family planning ("rhythm method")
- Barrier methods (i.e. condoms)
- Combined contraceptive pills
- Progestogen-only pills
- Coils (i.e. copper coil or Mirena)
- Progestogen injection
- Progestogen implant
- Surgery (i.e. sterilisation or vasectomy)

Emergency contraception is also available after unprotected intercourse. However, emergency contraception should not be relied upon as a regular method of contraception.

UK Medical Eligibility Criteria

The **Faculty of Sexual & Reproductive Healthcare** (**FSRH**) has **UK Medical Eligibility** (**UKMEC**) guidelines published in 2016 (updated in 2019) to categorise the risks of starting different methods of contraception in different individuals.

There are four levels, from least risk of most risk:
- **UKMEC 1**: No restriction in use (minimal risk)
- **UKMEC 2**: Benefits generally outweigh the risks
- **UKMEC 3**: Risks generally outweigh the benefits
- **UKMEC 4**: Unacceptable risk (typically this means the method is **contraindicated**)

Explaining Effectiveness

The different methods of contraception are not equally effective. The effectiveness is expressed as a percentage. For example, the combined oral contraceptive pill is 99% effective. The only method that is 100% effective is complete abstinence.

What 99% effective means is that if an **average person** used this method of contraception **correctly** with a **regular partner** for a **single year**, they would only have a 1% chance of pregnancy.

It is essential to distinguish between the effectiveness of **perfect use** and **typical use**. This is especially important with methods such as natural family planning, barrier contraception and the pill, where the effectiveness is very user-dependent. Long-acting methods such as the implant, coil and surgery are the most effective with typical use, as they are not dependent on the user to take regular action.

The **FSRH UKMEC guideline** (2016) provides data on the effectiveness of each method with perfect and typical use:

Method	Perfect Use	Typical Use
Natural Family Planning	95 - 99.6%	76%
Condoms	98%	82%
Combined oral contraceptive pill	> 99%	91%
Progestogen-only pill	> 99%	91%
Progestogen-only injection	> 99%	94%
Progestogen-only implant	> 99%	> 99%
Coils (i.e. copper coil or Mirena)	> 99%	> 99%
Surgery (i.e. sterilisation or vasectomy)	> 99%	> 99%

Specific Risk Factors

Exam questions frequently present an individual with specific risk factors and ask for the most suitable form of contraception for that person. It helps to remember key risk factors and their contraindications:
- **Breast cancer**: avoid any hormonal contraception and go for the copper coil or barrier methods
- **Cervical** or **endometrial cancer**: avoid the intrauterine system (i.e. Mirena coil)
- **Wilson's disease**: avoid the copper coil

There are specific risk factors that should make you avoid the **combined contraceptive pill** (UKMEC 4):
- Uncontrolled hypertension (particularly ≥160 / ≥100)
- Migraine with aura
- History of VTE
- Aged over 35 AND smoking more than 15 cigarettes per day
- Major surgery with prolonged immobility
- Vascular disease or stroke
- Ischaemic heart disease, cardiomyopathy or atrial fibrillation
- Liver cirrhosis and liver tumours
- Systemic lupus erythematosus and antiphospholipid syndrome

Older Women

There are some additional considerations in older and perimenopausal women:
- After the last period, contraception is required for 2 years in women under 50 and 1 year in women over 50
- **Hormone replacement therapy** does **not** prevent pregnancy, and added contraception is required
- The **combined contraceptive pill** can be used up to age 50 years, and can treat **perimenopausal symptoms**
- The **progestogen injection** (i.e. Depo-Provera) should be stopped before 50 years due to the risk of **osteoporosis**

Women that are **amenorrhoeic** (no periods) when taking **progestogen-only** contraception should continue until either:
- **FSH blood test** results are above 30 IU/L on two tests taken six weeks apart (continue contraception for 1 more year)
- 55 years of age

Choice of Contraception Under 20

When prescribing contraception to women under 20 years:
- **Combined** and **progestogen-only pills** are unaffected by younger age
- The **progestogen-only implant** is a good choice of **long-acting reversible contraception** (UK MEC 1)
- The **progestogen-only injection** is UK MEC 2 due to concerns about reduced **bone mineral density**
- **Coils** are UKMEC 2, as they may have a higher rate of expulsion

Contraception after Childbirth

Fertility is not considered to return until **21 days** after giving birth, and contraception is not required up to this point. The risk of pregnancy is very low before 21 days. After 21 days women are considered fertile, and will need contraception (including condoms for 7 days when starting the combined pill or 2 days for the progestogen-only pill).

Lactational amenorrhea is over 98% effective as contraception for up to 6 months after birth. Women must be **fully breastfeeding** and **amenorrhoeic** (no periods).

The **progestogen-only pill** and **implant** are considered safe in breastfeeding and can be started at any time after birth.

The **combined contraceptive pill** should be avoided in breastfeeding (UKMEC 4 before 6 weeks postpartum, UKMEC 2 after 6 weeks).

The **copper coil** or **intrauterine system** (e.g. Mirena) can be inserted either within 48 hours of birth or more than 4 weeks after birth (UKMEC 1), but not inserted between 48 hours and 4 weeks of birth (UKMEC 3).

TOM TIP: Remember that the combined pill should not be started before 6 weeks after childbirth in women that are breastfeeding. The progesterone-only pill or implant can be started any time after birth.

Barrier Methods

Barrier methods provide a **physical barrier** to semen entering the uterus and causing pregnancy. They are the only method that help protect against **sexually transmitted infections** (**STIs**). They are not 100% effective for contraception or preventing STIs.

Condoms

Condoms are about 98% effective with perfect use, but can be significantly less effective with typical use (82%). Standard condoms are made of **latex**. Using **oil-based lubricants** can damage latex condoms and make it more likely they will tear. **Polyurethane** condoms can be used in latex allergy.

Diaphragms and Cervical Caps

Diaphragms and **cervical caps** are silicone cups that fit over the cervix and prevent semen entering the uterus. The woman fits them before having sex, and leaves them in place for at least 6 hours after sex. They should be used with **spermicide gel** the further reduce the risk of pregnancy.

When used perfectly with spermicide, diaphragms and cervical caps are around 95% effective at preventing pregnancy. They offer little protection against STIs, and condoms need to be used for STI protection.

Dental Dams

Dental dams are used during oral sex to provide a barrier between the mouth and the vulva, vagina or anus. They are used to prevent infections that can be spread through oral sex, including:
- Chlamydia
- Gonorrhoea
- Herpes simplex 1 and 2
- HPV (human papillomavirus)
- E. coli
- Pubic lice
- Syphilis
- HIV

Combined Oral Contraceptive Pill

The combined oral contraceptive pill (**COCP**) contains a combination of **oestrogen** and **progesterone**. The combined pill is more than 99% effective with perfect use, but less effective with typical use (91%). The pill is licensed for use up to the age of 50 years.

Mechanism of Action

The COCP prevents pregnancy in three ways:
- **Preventing ovulation** (this is the primary mechanism of action)
- Progesterone thickens the cervical mucus
- Progesterone inhibits proliferation of the endometrium, reducing the chance of successful implantation

Oestrogen and **progesterone** have a **negative feedback** effect on the **hypothalamus** and **anterior pituitary**, suppressing the release of **GnRH**, **LH** and **FSH**. Without the effects of LH and FSH, ovulation does not occur. Pregnancy cannot happen without ovulation.

The lining of the endometrium is maintained in a stable state while taking the combined pill. When the pill is stopped the lining of the uterus breaks down and sheds. This leads to a "**withdrawal bleed**". This is not classed as a menstrual period as it is not part of the natural menstrual cycle. "**Breakthrough bleeding**" can occur with extended use without a pill-free period.

Types

There are two types of COCP to be aware of:
- **Monophasic pills** contain the same amount of hormone in each pill
- **Multiphasic pills** contain varying amounts of hormone to match the normal cyclical hormonal changes more closely

Everyday formulations (e.g. **Microgynon 30 ED**) are monophasic pills, but the pack contains seven **inactive pills**, making it easier for women to keep track by simply taking the pills in order every day.

Different formulations vary in the amount of oestrogen (**ethinylestradiol**) and the **type** of progesterone they contain. Examples of monophasic combined contraceptive pills are:
- **Microgynon** contains ethinylestradiol and **levonorgestrel**
- **Loestrin** contains ethinylestradiol and **norethisterone**
- **Cilest** contains ethinylestradiol and **norgestimate**
- **Yasmin** contains ethinylestradiol and **drospirenone**
- **Marvelon** contains ethinylestradiol and **desogestrel**

The NICE Clinical Knowledge Summaries (2020) recommend using a pill with **levonorgestrel** or **norethisterone** first-line (e.g. Microgynon or Leostrin). These choices have a lower risk of **venous thromboembolism**.

Yasmin and other COCPs containing **drospirenone** are considered first-line for **premenstrual syndrome**. Drospirenone has **anti-mineralocorticoid** and **anti-androgen** activity, and may help with symptoms of bloating, water retention and mood changes. **Continuous use** of the pill, as opposed to cyclical use, may be more effective for premenstrual syndrome.

Dianette and other COCPs containing **cyproterone acetate** (i.e. **co-cyprindiol**) can be considered in the treatment of **acne** and **hirsutism**. **Cyproterone acetate** has **anti-androgen** effects, helping to improve acne and hirsutism. The oestrogenic effects mean that co-cyprindiol has a 1.5 - 2 times greater risk of **venous thromboembolism** compared to the first-line combined pills (e.g. Microgynon). It is usually stopped three months after acne is controlled, due to the higher risk of VTE.

Regimes

The combined pill can be taken in different regimes to suit the individual. These regimes are equally safe and effective. Three common options are:
- 21 days on and 7 days off
- 63 days on (three packs) and 7 days off ("**tricycling**")
- Continuous use without a pill-free period

Side Effects and Risks

- **Unscheduled bleeding** is common in the first three months and should settle with time
- Breast pain and tenderness
- Mood changes and depression
- Headaches
- Hypertension
- Venous thromboembolism (the risk is much lower for the pill than pregnancy)
- Small increased risk of **breast** and **cervical** cancer, returning to normal ten years after stopping
- Small increased risk of myocardial infarction and stroke

Benefits

The benefits of the combined pill include:
- Effective contraception
- Rapid return of fertility after stopping
- Improvement in **premenstrual symptoms**, **menorrhagia** (heavy periods) and **dysmenorrhoea** (painful periods)
- Reduced risk of **endometrial**, **ovarian** and **colon** cancer
- Reduced risk of benign ovarian cysts

Contraindications

When starting any form of contraception, it is essential to consider the contraindications for the individual. There are specific risk factors that should make you avoid the **combined contraceptive pill** (**UKMEC 4**):
- Uncontrolled hypertension (particularly ≥160 / ≥100)
- Migraine with aura (risk of stroke)
- History of VTE
- Aged over 35 and smoking more than 15 cigarettes per day
- Major surgery with prolonged immobility
- Vascular disease or stroke
- Ischaemic heart disease, cardiomyopathy or atrial fibrillation
- Liver cirrhosis and liver tumours
- Systemic lupus erythematosus (SLE) and antiphospholipid syndrome

It is worth noting that a **BMI above 35** is **UKMEC 3** for the combined pill (risks generally outweigh the benefits).

TOM TIP: The UKMEC guidelines have helpful tables that allow you to compare risk factors quickly and assess which form of contraception is most suited to the individual. It is worth looking these up and getting familiar with them, then using them when counselling patients if required.

Starting the Pill

Start on the first day of the cycle (first day of the menstrual period). This offers protection straight away. No additional contraception is required if the pill is started up to day 5 of the menstrual cycle.

Starting **after day 5** of the menstrual cycle requires extra contraception (i.e. condoms) for the **first 7 days** of consistent pill use before they are protected from pregnancy. Ensure the woman is not already pregnant before starting the pill (i.e. they have been using alternative contraception reliably and consistently).

When switching between COCPs, finish one pack, then immediately start the new pill pack without the pill-free period.

When switching from a **traditional progesterone-only pill** (POP), they can switch at any time but **7 days** of extra contraception (i.e. condoms) is required. Ensure the woman is not already pregnant before switching (i.e. they have been using the POP reliably and consistently).

When switching from **desogestrel**, they can switch immediately, and no additional contraception is required. This differs from a traditional POP because desogestrel *inhibits ovulation*.

Consultation

There are several things to check and discuss when prescribing the combined pill:
- Different contraceptive options, including **long-acting reversible contraception** (LARC)
- Contraindications
- Adverse effects
- Instructions for taking the pill, including missed pills
- Factors that will impact the efficacy (e.g. diarrhoea and vomiting)
- Sexually transmitted infections (the pill is not protective)
- Safeguarding concerns (particularly in those under 16)

Screen for contraindications by discussing and documenting:
- Age
- Weight and height (BMI)
- Blood pressure
- Smoker or non-smoker
- Past medical history (particularly migraine, VTE, cancer, cardiovascular disease and SLE)
- Family history (particularly VTE and breast cancer)

Missed Pills

Missed pill rules are commonly tested in exams, either in MCQs or by having to council a patient in an OCSE scenario. It is worth understanding the theory as this makes it easier to work out what to do. In reality, always double-check the rules with guidelines or product literature to make sure you get it right.

The best way to understand the rules is to consider that *theoretically* women will be protected if they perfectly take the pill in a cycle of 7 days on, 7 days off. This will prevent ovulation.

Missing one pill is when the pill is **more than 24 hours late** (48 hours since the last pill was taken).

Missing one pill (less than 72 hours since the last pill was taken):
- Take the missed pill as soon as possible (even if this means taking two pills on the same day)
- No extra protection is required provided other pills before and after are taken correctly

Missing more than one pill (more than 72 hours since the last pill was taken):
- Take the most recent missed pill as soon as possible (even if this means taking two pills on the same day)
- Additional contraception (i.e. condoms) is needed until they have taken the pill regularly for 7 days straight
- If day 1 - 7 of the packet they need emergency contraception if they have had unprotected sex
- If day 8 - 14 of the pack (and day 1 - 7 was fully compliant) then no emergency contraception is required
- If day 15 - 21 of the pack (and day 1 - 14 was fully compliant) then no emergency contraception is needed. They should go back-to-back with their next pack of pills and skip the pill-free period.

Theoretically, additional contraception is not required if more than one pill is missed between day 8 - 21 (week 2 or 3) of the pill packet and they otherwise take the pills correctly, although it is recommended for extra precaution.

Final Considerations

Vomiting, **diarrhoea** and certain **medications** (e.g. rifampicin) can all reduce the effectiveness of the pill, and additional contraception may be required. A day of vomiting or diarrhoea is classed as a "missed pill" day, as the illness may affect the absorption.

NICE Clinical Knowledge Summaries (January 2019) recommend stopping the combined pill **four weeks** before a **major operation** (lasting more than 30 minutes), or any operation or procedure that requires the lower limb to be immobilised. This is to reduce the risk of thrombosis.

Progestogen-Only Pill

The progestogen-only pill (**POP**) is a type of contraceptive pill that only contains progesterone. The POP is taken continuously, unlike the cyclical combined pills. It is more than 99% effective with perfect use, but less effective with typical use (91%).

The progestogen-only pill has far fewer contraindications and risks compared with the combined pill. The only **UKMEC 4** criteria for the POP is **active breast cancer**.

Types

There are two types of POP to remember:
- **Traditional** progestogen-only pill (e.g. Norgeston or Noriday)
- **Desogestrel-only pill** (e.g. Cerazette)

The **traditional progestogen-only pill** cannot be delayed by more than **3 hours**. Taking the pill more than 3 hours late is considered a "missed pill".

The **desogestrel-only pill** can be taken up to 12 hours late and still be effective. Taking the pill more than 12 hours late is considered a "missed pill".

Mechanism of Action

Traditional progestogen-only pills work mainly by:
- Thickening the cervical mucus
- Altering the endometrium and making it less accepting of implantation
- Reducing ciliary action in the fallopian tubes

Desogestrel works mainly by:
- **Inhibiting ovulation**
- Thickening the cervical mucus
- Altering the endometrium
- Reducing ciliary action in the fallopian tubes

Starting the Pill

Starting the POP on day 1 to 5 of the menstrual cycle means the woman is protected immediately.

It can be started at other times of the cycle provided pregnancy can be excluded. Additional contraception is required for **48 hours**. It takes 48 hours for the cervical mucus to thicken enough to prevent sperm entering the uterus.

The POP can be started even if there is a risk of pregnancy, as it is not known to be harmful in pregnancy. However, the woman should do a pregnancy test 3 weeks after the last unprotected intercourse. Emergency contraception before starting the pill may be considered if required.

TOM TIP: It takes 48 hours before the progestogen-only pill thickens the cervical mucus enough to prevent sperm entering the uterus, protecting against pregnancy. The combined pill takes seven days before the woman is protected from pregnancy, as it works by inhibiting ovulation rather than thickening the cervical mucus. Therefore, additional contraception is required for 48 hours with the POP and seven days with the COCP when starting after day 5 of the menstrual cycle. Both can be started within the first 5 days of the menstrual cycle and work immediately, as it is very unlikely a woman will ovulate this early in the cycle.

Switching Pills

Switching between POPs
POPs can be switched immediately without any need for extra contraception.

Switching from a COCP to a POP
When switching from a COCP to a POP, the directions depend on what point they are in the COCP pill packet. The best time to change is on day 1 to 7 of the hormone-free period after finishing the COCP pack, in which case no additional contraception is required.

Sometimes it is essential to switch immediately, for example, if they develop migraines with aura. If they have not had sex since finishing the COCP pack, they can switch straight away but need to use extra contraception (i.e. condoms) for the first 48 hours of the POP.

If they have had sex since completing the last pack of combined pills, they need to have completed at least seven consecutive days of the combined pill before switching, then use extra contraception for 48 hours. If this is not possible, emergency contraception may need to be considered.

Side Effects and Risks

Changes to the bleeding schedule is one of the primary adverse effects of the progestogen-only pill. **Unscheduled bleeding** is common in the first three months and often settles after that. Where the irregular bleeding is persistent (for longer than 3 months), other causes need to be excluded (e.g. STIs, pregnancy or cancer).

Approximately:
- 20% have no bleeding (**amenorrhoea**)
- 40% have regular bleeding
- 40% have irregular, prolonged or troublesome bleeding

Other side effects include:
- Breast tenderness
- Headaches
- Acne

There is also an increased risk of:
- Ovarian cysts
- Small risk of ectopic pregnancy with traditional POPs (not desogestrel) due to reduce ciliary action in the tubes
- Minimal increased risk of breast cancer, returning to normal ten years after stopping

TOM TIP: The bleeding pattern that a woman will experience with progestogen-only contraception (the pill, implant or injection) is unpredictable. To make it simple to remember I round the risks into thirds, with a third having lighter, less regular or no bleeding, a third having normal bleeding and a third having unscheduled, heavier or more prolonged bleeding. It is not possible to predict how individuals will respond. Irregular or troublesome bleeding often settles after three months, so it may be worth persisting.

Missed Pills

A pill is classed as "missed" if it is:
- More than **3 hours** late for a **traditional POP** (more than 26 hours after the last pill)
- More than **12 hours** late for the **desogestrel POP** (more than 36 hours after the last pill)

The instructions are to take a pill as soon as possible, continue with the next pill at the usual time (even if this means taking two in 24 hours) and use extra contraception for the next 48 hours of regular use. **Emergency contraception** is required if they have had sex since missing the pill or within 48 hours of restarting the regular pills.

Episodes of **diarrhoea** or **vomiting** are managed as "missed pills". Extra contraception (i.e. condoms) is required until 48 hours after the diarrhoea and vomiting settle.

Progestogen-Only Injection

The progestogen-only injection is also known as **depot medroxyprogesterone acetate** (**DMPA**). You will see it listed as "DMPA" in the UK MEC guidelines. It is given at 12 to 13 week intervals as an **intramuscular** or **subcutaneous** injection of **medroxyprogesterone acetate** (a type of **progestin**).

The DMPA is more than 99% effective with perfect use, but less effective with typical use (94%). It is less effective with typical use because women may forget to book in for an injection every 12 to 13 weeks.

It can take 12 months for fertility to return after stopping the injections, making it less suitable for women who may wish to get pregnant in the near term.

There are two versions commonly used in the UK, all containing **medroxyprogesterone acetate**:
- **Depo-Provera**: given by **intramuscular** injection
- **Sayana Press**: a **subcutaneous** injection device that can be **self-injected** by the patient

Noristerat is an alternative to the DMPA that contains **norethisterone** and works for eight weeks. This is usually used as a short term interim contraception (e.g. after the partner has a vasectomy) rather than a long term solution.

Contraindications

UK MEC 4
- Active breast cancer

UK MEC 3
- Ischaemic heart disease and stroke
- Unexplained vaginal bleeding
- Severe liver cirrhosis
- Liver cancer

The DMPA can cause **osteoporosis**. This is something to consider in older women and patients on steroids for asthma or inflammatory conditions. It is UK MEC 2 in women over 45 years, and women should generally switch to an alternative by age 50 years.

Mechanism

The main action of the depot injection is to **inhibit ovulation**. It does this by inhibiting **FSH** secretion by the **pituitary gland**, preventing the development of **follicles** in the ovaries.

Additionally, the depot injection works by:
- Thickening cervical mucus
- Altering the endometrium and making it less accepting of implantation

Timing the Injection

Starting on day 1 to 5 of the menstrual cycle offers immediate protection, and no extra contraception is required.

Starting after day 5 of the menstrual cycle requires **seven days** of extra contraception (e.g. condoms) before the injection becomes reliably effective.

Women need to have injections every 12 - 13 weeks. Delaying past 13 weeks creates a risk of pregnancy. The FSRH guidelines say it can be given as early as 10 weeks and as late as 14 weeks after the last injection where necessary, but this is unlicensed.

Side Effects and Risks

Changes to the bleeding schedule is one of the primary considerations with progestogen-only contraception. Bleeding often becomes more irregular, and in some women, it may be heavier and last longer. This is usually temporary, and after a year of regular use, most women will stop bleeding altogether (amenorrhoea). It is not possible to predict how individuals will respond.

Other side effects include:
- Weight gain
- Acne
- Reduced libido
- Mood changes
- Headaches
- Flushes
- Hair loss (**alopecia**)
- Skin reactions at injection sites

Reduced bone mineral density (**osteoporosis**) is an important side effect of the depot injection. **Oestrogen** helps maintain **bone mineral density** in women, and is mainly produced by the **follicles** in the **ovaries**. Suppressing the development of **follicles** reduces the amount of **oestrogen** produced, and this can lead to decreased bone mineral density.

The depot injection may be associated with a very small increased risk of **breast** and **cervical cancer**.

TOM TIP: The two side effects that are unique to the progestogen injection are weight gain and osteoporosis. These adverse effects are not associated with any other forms of contraception, making them a useful fact for examiners to ask about in exams.

Problematic Bleeding

Irregular bleeding can occur, particularly in the first six months. This often settles with time. The longer the woman is taking the injection, the more likely she is to have no bleeding (amenorrhoea). Alternative causes need to be excluded where problematic bleeding continues, including a **sexual health screen**, **pregnancy test** and ensuring **cervical screening** is up to date.

The FSRH guidelines suggest taking the **combined oral contraceptive pill** (COCP) in addition to the injection for three months when problematic bleeding occurs, to help settle the bleeding. Another option is a short course (5 days) of mefenamic acid to halt the bleeding.

Potential Benefits

There are several possible benefits of the injection, with evidence that it:
- Improves **dysmenorrhoea** (painful periods)
- Improves **endometriosis**-related symptoms
- Reduces the risk of **ovarian** and **endometrial cancer**
- Reduces the severity of **sickle cell crisis** in patients with sickle cell anaemia

Progestogen-Only Implant

The progestogen-only implant is a small (4cm) flexible plastic rod that is placed in the upper arm, beneath the skin and above the subcutaneous fat. It slowly releases progestogen into the systemic circulation. It lasts for **three years** and then needs replacing.

The progestogen-only implant is more than 99% effective with perfect and typical use. Once in place, there is no room for user error. It needs to be replaced every three years to remain effective.

The progestogen-only implant has very few contraindications and risks. The only UKMEC 4 criteria for the implant is **active breast cancer**.

Nexplanon is the implant used in the UK. It contains 68mg of **etonogestrel**. It is licensed for use between the ages of 18 and 40 years.

Mechanism

The progestogen-only implant works by:
- Inhibiting ovulation
- Thickening cervical mucus
- Altering the endometrium and making it less accepting of implantation

Insertion and Removal

Inserting the implant on day 1 to 5 of the menstrual cycle provides immediate protection. Insertion after day 5 of the menstrual cycle requires **seven days** of extra contraception (e.g. condoms), similar to the injection.

Specific qualifications are required to **insert** the implant. It is inserted one-third the way up the upper arm, on the medial side. Local anaesthetic (lidocaine) is used prior to inserting the implant. A specially designed device is used to insert the implant horizontally, beneath the skin and above the subcutaneous fat. It should be palpable immediately after insertion. Pressing on one end of the implant should make the other end pop upwards against the skin.

Specific qualifications are also required to **remove** the implant. Lidocaine is used as a local anaesthetic. The device is located, and a small incision is made in the skin at one end. The device is removed using pressure on the other end, or forceps. Contraception is required immediately after it has been removed (but not immediately before).

Benefits

- Effective and reliable contraception
- It can improve **dysmenorrhoea** (painful menstruation)
- It can make periods lighter or stop all together
- No need to remember to take pills (just remember to change the device every three years)
- It does not cause weight gain (unlike the depo injection)
- No effect on bone mineral density (unlike the depo injection)
- No increase in thrombosis risk (unlike the COCP)
- No restrictions for use in obese patients (unlike the COCP)

Drawbacks

Several factors may limit the appeal of the implant:
- It requires a minor operation with a local anaesthetic to insert and remove the device
- It can lead to worsening of acne
- There is no protection against sexually transmitted infections
- It can cause problematic bleeding
- Implants can be bent or fractured
- Implants can become impalpable or deeply implanted, leading to investigations and additional management

Rarely the implant can become impalpable or deeply implanted. Women are advised to palpate the implant occasionally, and if it becomes impalpable, extra contraception is required until it is located. An **ultrasound** or **xray** may be required to locate an impalpable implant. They may need referral to a specialist removal centre. The manufacturer of Nexplanon adds **barium sulphate** to make it **radio-opaque** so that it can be seen on xrays.

In very rare cases there are reports of devices entering blood vessels and migrating through the body, including to the lungs. If the implant cannot be located even after an ultrasound scan, a chest xray may be considered to identify an implant in a pulmonary artery.

Bleeding Pattern

The FSRH guideline on the implant (2014) state approximately:
- 1/3 have infrequent bleeding
- 1/4 have frequent or prolonged bleeding
- 1/5 have no bleeding
- The remainder have normal regular bleeds

Problematic bleeding is managed similarly to the progestogen-only implant. The FSRH guidelines suggest the **combined oral contraceptive pill** (COCP) in addition to the implant for three months when problematic bleeding occurs, to help settle the bleeding (provided there are no contraindications).

Coils

Coils are devices inserted into the uterus that provide contraception. They are a form of **long-acting reversible contraception**. Once fitted, they work for a long time. Removing the device restores fertility.

There are two types of **intrauterine device** (**IUD**):
- **Copper coil** (**Cu-IUD**): contains copper and creates a hostile environment for pregnancy
- **Levonorgestrel intrauterine system** (**LNG-IUS**): contains progestogen that is slowly released into the uterus

Both types of coil are more than 99% effective when properly inserted. Fertility returns immediately after removal of an intrauterine device.

TOM TIP: Often, the two types of coil are referred to as IUD and IUS. The intrauterine device (IUD) refers to the copper coil, and the intrauterine system (IUS) refers to the levonorgestrel (e.g. Mirena) coil. The copper coil is just a "device", whereas the hormones in the Mirena make it a "system".

Contraindications

- Pelvic inflammatory disease or infection
- Immunosuppression
- Pregnancy
- Unexplained bleeding
- Pelvic cancer
- Uterine cavity distortion (e.g. by fibroids)

Insertion and Removal

Insertion
In women at increased risk of sexually transmitted infections (e.g. under 25 years old), screening for chlamydia and gonorrhoea is performed before insertion of a coil.

Specific qualifications are required to insert the implant. A bimanual is performed before the procedure to check the position and size of the uterus. A speculum is inserted, and specialised equipment is used to fit the device. Forceps can be used to stabilise the cervix while the device is inserted. Blood pressure and heart rate are recorded before and after insertion.

There may be some temporary crampy, period-like pain after insertion. NSAIDs may be used to help with discomfort after the procedure. Women need to be seen 3 to 6 weeks after insertion to check the threads. They should be taught to feel the strings to ensure the coil remains in place.

Risks relating to the insertion of the coil include:
- Bleeding
- Pain on insertion
- Vasovagal reactions (dizziness, bradycardia and arrhythmias)
- Uterine perforation (1 in 1000, higher in breastfeeding women)
- Pelvic inflammatory disease (particularly in the first 20 days)
- The expulsion rate is highest in the first three months

Removal

Before the coil is removed, women need to abstain from sex or use condoms for 7 days, or there is a risk of pregnancy. The strings are located and slowly pulled to remove the device.

Non-Visible Threads

When the coil threads cannot be seen or palpated, three things need to be excluded:
- Expulsion
- Pregnancy
- Uterine perforation

Extra contraception (i.e. condoms) is required until the coil is located.

The initial investigation is an **ultrasound**. An abdominal and pelvic **xray** can be used to look for a coil elsewhere in the abdomen or peritoneal cavity after a uterine perforation. **Hysteroscopy** or **laparoscopic surgery** may be required depending on the location of the coil.

Copper Coil

The copper coil (**IUD**) is a form of **long-acting reversible contraception** licensed for 5 - 10 years after insertion (depending on the device). It can also be used as **emergency contraception**, inserted up to 5 days after an episode of unprotected intercourse. It is notably contraindicated in **Wilson's disease**.

Mechanism
Copper is toxic to the ovum and sperm. It also alters the endometrium and makes it less accepting of implantation.

Benefits
- Reliable contraception
- It can be inserted at any time in the menstrual cycle and is effective immediately
- It contains no hormones, so it is safe for women at risk of VTE or with a history of hormone-related cancers
- It may reduce the risk of endometrial and cervical cancer

Drawbacks
- A procedure is required to insert and remove the coil, with associated risks
- It can cause heavy or intermenstrual bleeding (this often settles)
- Some women experience pelvic pain
- It does not protect against sexually transmitted infections
- Increased risk of ectopic pregnancies
- Intrauterine devices can occasionally fall out (around 5%)

TOM TIP: The copper coil is contraindicated in Wilson's disease. Wilson's disease is a condition where there is excessive accumulation of copper in the body and tissues. Examiners like to add questions on this, as it requires knowledge of the copper coil and Wilson's disease.

Levonorgestrel Intrauterine System

There are four types of IUS you may come across, all containing **levonorgestrel**:
- **Mirena**: effective for 5 years for contraception, and also licensed for menorrhagia and HRT
- **Levosert**: effective for 5 years, and also licensed for menorrhagia
- **Kyleena**: effective for 5 years
- **Jaydess**: effective for 3 years

TOM TIP: *The IUS to remember is the Mirena coil. It is commonly used for contraception, menorrhagia and endometrial protection for women on HRT. It is licensed for 5 years for contraception, but only 4 years for HRT.*

The **LNG-IUS** works by releasing **levonorgestrel** (progestogen) into the local area:
- Thickening cervical mucus
- Altering the endometrium and making it less accepting of implantation
- Inhibiting ovulation in a small number of women

The **LNG-IUS** can be inserted up to day 7 of the menstrual cycle without a need for additional contraception. If it is inserted after day 7, pregnancy needs to be reasonably excluded, and extra protection (i.e. condoms) is required for 7 days.

Benefits
- It can make periods lighter or stop altogether
- It may improve dysmenorrhoea or pelvic pain related to endometriosis
- No effect on bone mineral density (unlike the depo injection)
- No increase in thrombosis risk (unlike the COCP)
- No restrictions for use in obese patients (unlike the COCP)
- The Mirena has additional uses (i.e. HRT and menorrhagia)

Drawbacks
- A procedure is required to insert and remove the coil, with associated risks
- It can cause spotting or irregular bleeding
- Some women experience pelvic pain
- It does not protect against sexually transmitted infections
- Increased risk of ectopic pregnancies
- Increased incidence of ovarian cysts
- There can be systemic absorption causing side effects of acne, headaches, or breast tenderness
- Intrauterine devices can occasionally fall out (around 5%)

Problematic Bleeding
Irregular bleeding can occur, particularly in the first six months. This usually settles with time. Alternative causes need to be excluded where problematic bleeding continues, including a **sexual health screen**, **pregnancy test** and ensuring **cervical screening** is up to date.

The FSRH guidelines suggest taking the **combined oral contraceptive pill** (COCP) in addition to the **LNG-IUS** for three months when problematic bleeding occurs, to help settle the bleeding.

Actinomyces-Like Organisms on Smears

Actinomyces-like organisms (**ALOs**) are often discovered incidentally during smear tests in women with an **intrauterine device** (coil). This does not require treatment unless the patient is symptomatic. Where the woman is symptomatic (e.g. pelvic pain or abnormal bleeding), removal of the intrauterine device may be considered.

Emergency Contraception

Emergency contraception can be used after episodes of **unprotected sexual intercourse** (**UPSI**). This includes situations where the contraceptive method is not protective, such as damaged condoms or multiple missed pills.

There are three options for emergency contraception:
- **Levonorgestrel** should be taken within 72 hours of UPSI
- **Ulipristal** should be taken within 120 hours of UPSI
- **Copper coil** can be inserted within 5 days of UPSI, or within 5 days of the estimated date of ovulation

The copper coil is the most effective. It is also not affected by **BMI**, **enzyme-inducing drugs** or **malabsorption**, all of which can significantly reduce the effectiveness of oral methods.

With oral emergency contraception, the sooner it is taken, the more effective it is. Oral emergency contraception is unlikely to be effective after ovulation has occurred; however, it is offered after UPSI on any day of the menstrual cycle. The woman needs to take a pregnancy test if her period is delayed.

Oral emergency contraception does not protect against further episodes of UPSI. The FSRH guidelines (2017) state that both levonorgestrel and ulipristal can be used more than once in a menstrual cycle.

Other things to consider when starting emergency contraception:
- Reassure about confidentiality
- Sexually transmitted infections
- Future contraception plans
- Safeguarding, rape and abuse

Intrauterine Device

The copper coil can be used as an emergency contraception up to 5 days after unprotected intercourse, or within 5 days after the earliest **estimated date of ovulation**. Ovulation occurs 14 days before the end of the cycle, so if a woman's shortest cycle length is 28 days, the earliest estimated date of ovulation is day 14. It would be day 12 for a 26-day cycle, or day 16 for a 30-day cycle.

The copper coil is toxic to the ovum and sperm, and also inhibits implantation. It is the most effective emergency contraception, being over 99% effective. The FSRH guidelines (2017) advised offering the copper coil first-line for emergency contraception.

Insertion may lead to **pelvic inflammatory disease**, particularly in women that are at high risk of sexually transmitted infections. Consider empirical treatment of pelvic infections where the risk is high.

The coil should be kept in until at least the next period, after which it can be removed. Alternatively, it can be left in long-term as contraception.

Levonorgestrel

Levonorgestrel is a type of **progestogen**. It works by preventing or delaying ovulation. It is the same hormone found in the intrauterine system (hormonal coil). It is not known to be harmful if pregnancy does occur.

The **combined pill** or **progestogen-only pill** can be started **immediately** after taking levonorgestrel. Extra contraception (i.e. condoms) is required for the first 7 days of the combined pill or the first 2 days of the progestogen-only pill.

Levonorgestrel is licensed for use up to 72 hours post intercourse. The dose listed in the BNF is:
- 1.5mg as a single dose
- 3mg as a single dose in women above 70kg or BMI above 26

Nausea and vomiting are common side effects. If vomiting occurs within 3 hours of taking the pill, the dose should be repeated.

Other side effects include:
- Spotting and changes to the next menstrual period
- Diarrhoea
- Breast tenderness
- Dizziness
- Depressed mood

Levonorgestrel is not known to be harmful when breastfeeding, and breastfeeding can continue (unlikely ulipristal). The NICE CKS advise that breastfeeding is avoided for 8 hours after taking the dose to reduce the exposure to the infant.

Ulipristal

Ulipristal acetate is a **selective progesterone receptor modulator** (**SERM**) that works by delaying ovulation. The common brand name is **EllaOne**. It is more effective than levonorgestrel. It is not known to be harmful if pregnancy does occur; however, there is limited data on this.

Wait **5 days** before starting the **combined pill** or **progestogen-only pill** after taking ulipristal. Extra contraception (ie. condoms) is required for the first 7 days of the combined pill or the first 2 days of the progestogen-only pill.

It is given as a single dose (30mg) to prevent pregnancy after unprotected intercourse. Ulipristal is licensed for use up to 120 hours after intercourse.

Nausea and vomiting are common side effects. If vomiting occurs within 3 hours of taking the pill, the dose should be repeated.

Other side effects include:
- Spotting and changes to the next menstrual period
- Abdominal or pelvic pain
- Back pain
- Mood changes
- Headache
- Dizziness
- Breast tenderness

There are several notably restrictions with ulipristal:
- Breastfeeding should be avoided for 1 week after taking ulipristal (milk should be expressed and discarded)
- Ulipristal should be avoided in patients with **severe asthma**

Sterilisation

Sterilisation procedures are permanent surgical interventions to prevent conception. It is essential to thoroughly counsel patients about the permanence of the procedure, and ensure they have made a fully informed decision. Sterilisation does not protect against sexually transmitted infections.

The NHS does not provide **reversal** procedures. Private reversal procedures are available, but the success rate is low. Therefore, sterilisation should be considered permanent.

Tubal Occlusion

The **female sterilisation** procedure is called **tubal occlusion**. This is typically performed by **laparoscopy** under a **general anaesthesic**, with occlusion of the tubes using "**Filshie clips**". Alternatively, the fallopian types can be tied and cut, or removed altogether. This can be done as an **elective procedure**, or during a **caesarean section**.

The procedure works by preventing the **ovum** (egg) travelling from the ovary to the uterus along the fallopian tube. This means the ovum and sperm will not meet, and pregnancy cannot occur.

The procedure is more than 99% effective (1 in 200 failure rate). Alternative contraception is required until the next menstrual period, as an ovum may have already reached the uterus during that cycle, ready for fertilisation.

Vasectomy

The **male sterilisation** procedure is called a **vasectomy**. This involves cutting the **vas deferens**, preventing sperm travelling from the testes to join the ejaculated fluid. This prevents sperm being released into the vagina, preventing pregnancy. It is more than 99% effective (1 in 2000 failure rate).

The procedure is performed under **local anaesthetic** and is relatively quick (15 - 20 minutes). This makes it a less invasive procedure than female sterilisation and often a better option for couples that are considering permanent means of contraception.

Alternative contraception is required for two months after the procedure. Testing of the semen to confirm the absence of sperm is necessary before it can be relied upon for contraception. Semen testing is usually carried out around 12 weeks after the procedure, as it takes time for sperm that are still in the tubes to be cleared. A second semen analysis may be required for confirmation.

Consent to Contraception

Where you are concerned or unsure about the law, you can talk to a senior or your medical defence organisation. This book gives an overview to help with your exam preparation, and cannot be used as advice about the law.

A person is recognised as an adult with full autonomy to make decisions about their health when they turn 18 years. 16 and 17-year-olds can also make independent decisions about their health, but if they refuse treatment, this can be overruled in certain situations by parents, people with parental responsibility or the court.

Children under 16 can make treatment decisions, but only if they are deemed to have **Gillick competence**. There is no lower limit to the age where children can make decisions about their health; however, it is unusual for consent to be taken from someone under 13.

The way this knowledge is usually tested in exams relates to girls under 16 years seeking contraception from their GP. This is the scenario that established "**Gillick competence**" and "**Frazer guidelines**" in the first place.

Gillick Competence

Gillick competence refers to a judgement about whether the understanding and intelligence of the child is sufficient to consent to treatment. Gillick competence needs to be assessed on a **decision by decision basis**, checking whether the child understands the implications of the treatment.

Consent needs to be given **voluntarily**. When prescribing contraception to children under 16 years, it is essential to assess for **coercion** or **pressure**, for example, coercion by an older partner. This might raise **safeguarding concerns**.

Frazer Guidelines

The Frazer guidelines are specific guidelines for providing contraception to patients under 16 years **without** having parental input and consent. The **House of Lords** established these guidelines in 1985. To follow the guidelines, they need to meet the following criteria:
1. They are mature and intelligent enough to understand the treatment
2. They can't be persuaded to discuss it with their parents or let the health professional discuss it
3. They are likely to have intercourse regardless of treatment
4. Their physical or mental health is likely to suffer without treatment
5. Treatment is in their best interest

Children should be encouraged to inform their parents, but if they decline and meet the criteria for Gillick competence and the Frazer guidelines, confidentiality can be kept.

Safeguarding When Providing Contraception

It is essential to explore whether there is any possibility of abuse or exploitation. When this is present, confidentiality may need to be broken. Where the child is not deemed to be Gillick competent, and the child is at risk of harm, this should be escalated as a safeguarding concern.

Children under 13 cannot give consent for sexual activity. All intercourse in children under 13 years should be escalated as a safeguarding concern to a senior or designated child protection doctor for further action.

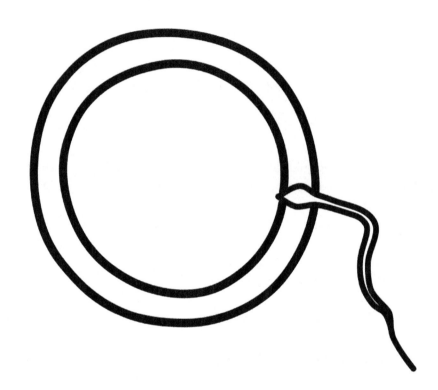

FERTILITY

6.1	Infertility	125
6.2	Male Factor Infertility	127
6.3	In Vitro Fertilisation	130
6.4	Ovarian Hyperstimulation Syndrome	132

Infertility

85% will conceive within a year of regular unprotected sex. 1 in 7 couples will struggle to conceive naturally.

Investigation and referral for infertility should be initiated after the couple has been trying to conceive without success for **12 months**. This can be reduced to 6 months if the woman is older than 35, as her ovarian stores are likely to be already reduced and time is more precious.

Causes

- Sperm problems (30%)
- Ovulation problems (25%)
- Tubal problems (15%)
- Uterine problems (10%)
- Unexplained (20%)

40% of infertile couples have a mix of male and female factors.

General Advice

There is some general lifestyle advice for couples trying to get pregnant:
- The woman should be taking 400mcg folic acid daily
- Aim for a healthy BMI
- Avoid smoking and drinking excessive alcohol
- Reduce stress as this may negatively affect libido and the relationship
- Aim for intercourse every 2 - 3 days
- Avoid timed intercourse

Timed intercourse to coincide with ovulation is not necessary or recommended. It can lead to increased stress and pressure in the relationship.

Investigations

Initial investigations, often performed in primary care:
- **Body mass index** (**BMI**) (low could indicate **anovulation**, high could indicate **PCOS**)
- Chlamydia screening
- Semen analysis
- Female hormonal testing (see below)
- Rubella immunity in the mother

Female hormone testing involves:
- **Serum LH** and **FSH** on **day 2 to 5** of the cycle
- **Serum progesterone** on **day 21** of the cycle (or 7 days before the end of the cycle if not a 28-day cycle).
- **Anti-Mullerian hormone**
- **Thyroid function tests** when symptoms are suggestive
- **Prolactin** (hyperprolactinaemia is a cause of anovulation) when symptoms of **galactorrhea** or **amenorrhoea**

High FSH suggests poor **ovarian reserve** (the number of **follicles** that the woman has left in her **ovaries**). The pituitary gland is producing extra FSH in an attempt to stimulate follicular development.

High LH may suggest **polycystic ovarian syndrome** (**PCOS**).

A rise in **progesterone** on day 21 indicates that **ovulation** has occurred, and the **corpus luteum** has formed and started secreting progesterone.

Anti-Mullerian hormone can be measured at any time during the cycle and is the most accurate marker of **ovarian reserve**. It is released by the **granulosa cells** in the follicles and falls as the eggs are depleted. A high level indicates a good **ovarian reserve**.

Further investigations, often performed in secondary care:
- **Ultrasound pelvis** to look for polycystic ovaries or any structural abnormalities in the uterus
- **Hysterosalpingogram** to look at the patency of the fallopian tubes
- **Laparoscopy and dye test** to look at the patency of the fallopian tubes, adhesions and endometriosis

Hysterosalpingogram

A hysterosalpingogram is a type of scan used to assess the shape of the uterus and the patency of the fallopian tubes. Not only does it help with diagnosis, but it also has therapeutic benefit. It seems to increase the rate of conception without any other intervention. **Tubal cannulation** under xray guidance can be performed during the procedure to open up the tubes.

A small tube is inserted into the cervix. A **contrast medium** is injected through the tube and fills the **uterine cavity** and **fallopian tubes**. Xray images are taken, and the contrast shows up on the xray giving an outline of the uterus and tubes. If the dye does not fill one of the tubes, this will be seen on an xray and suggests a tubal obstruction.

There is a risk of infection with the procedure, and often antibiotics are given prophylactically for patients with dilated tubes or a history of pelvic infection. Screening for **chlamydia** and **gonorrhoea** should be done before the procedure.

Laparoscopy and Dye Test

The patient is admitted for laparoscopy. During the procedure, dye is injected into the uterus and should be seen entering the fallopian tubes and spilling out at the ends of the tubes. This will not be seen when there is tubal obstruction. During laparoscopy, the surgeon can also assess for endometriosis or pelvic adhesions, and treat these.

Management of Anovulation

The options when **anovulation** is the cause of infertility include:
- **Weight loss** for overweight patients with PCOS can restore ovulation
- **Clomifene** may be used to stimulate ovulation
- **Letrozole** may be used instead of clomifene to stimulate ovulation (**aromatase inhibitor** with **anti-oestrogen** effects)
- **Gonadotropins** may be used to stimulate ovulation in women resistant to clomifene
- **Ovarian drilling** may be used in polycystic ovarian syndrome
- **Metformin** may be used when there is **insulin insensitivity** and **obesity** (usually associated with **PCOS**)

Clomifene is an **anti-oestrogen** (a **selective oestrogen receptor modulator**). It is given daily between days 2 to 6 of the menstrual cycle. It stops the negative feedback of **oestrogen** on the **hypothalamus**, resulting in a greater release of **GnRH** and subsequently **FSH** and **LH**.

Ovarian drilling involves **laparoscopic surgery**. The surgeon punctures multiple holes in the ovaries using **diathermy** or **laser therapy**. This can improve the woman's hormonal profile and result in regular ovulation and fertility.

Management of Tubal Factors

The options for women with alterations to the fallopian tubes that prevent the ovum from reaching the sperm and uterus include:
- Tubal cannulation during a hysterosalpingogram
- Laparoscopy to remove adhesions or endometriosis
- In vitro fertilisation (IVF)

Management of Uterine Factors

Surgery may be used to correct polyps, adhesions or structural abnormalities affecting fertility.

Management of Sperm Problems

Surgical sperm retrieval is used when there is a blockage somewhere along the vas deferens preventing sperm from reaching the ejaculated semen. A needle and syringe is used to collect sperm directly from the **epididymis** through the scrotum.

Surgical correction of an obstruction in the vas deferens may restore male fertility.

Intra-uterine insemination involves collecting and separating out high-quality sperm, then injecting them directly into the uterus to give them the best chance of success. It is unclear whether this is any better than normal intercourse.

Intracytoplasmic sperm injection (**ICSI**) involves injecting sperm directly into the cytoplasm of an egg. These fertilised eggs become embryos, and are injected into the uterus of the woman. This is useful when there are significant motility issues, a very low sperm count and other issues with the sperm.

Donor insemination with sperm from a donor is another option for male factor infertility.

Male Factor Infertility

Semen analysis is used to examine the **quantity** and **quality** of the **semen** and **sperm**. It assesses for **male factor infertility**.

Providing a Sample

Men should be given clear instructions for providing a sample:
- Abstain from ejaculation for at least 3 days and at most 7 days
- Avoid hot baths, sauna and tight underwear during the lead up to providing a sample

- Attempt to catch the full sample
- Deliver the sample to the lab within 1 hour of ejaculation
- Keep the sample warm (e.g. in underwear) before delivery

Factors Affecting Semen Analysis

Several factors may affect the results of semen analysis:

- Hot baths
- Tight underwear
- Smoking
- Alcohol
- Raised BMI
- Caffeine

A repeat sample is indicated after 3 months in borderline results or earlier (2 - 4 weeks) with very abnormal results.

Results

Normal results indicated by the World Health Organisation are:
- **Semen volume** (more than 1.5ml)
- **Semen pH** (greater than 7.2)
- **Concentration** of sperm (more than 15 million per ml)
- **Total number** of sperm (more than 39 million per sample)
- **Motility** of sperm (more than 40% of sperm are mobile)
- **Vitality** of sperm (more than 58% of sperm are active)
- **Percentage** of normal sperm (more than 4%)

Polyspermia (or polyzoospermia) refers to a high number of sperm in the semen sample (more than 250 million per ml).

Normospermia (or normozoospermia) refers to normal characteristics of the sperm in the semen sample.

Oligospermia (or oligozoospermia) is a reduced number of sperm in the semen sample. It is classified as:
- Mild oligospermia (10 to 15 million / ml)
- Moderate oligospermia (5 to 10 million / ml)
- Severe oligospermia (less than 5 million / ml)

Cryptozoospermia refers to very few sperm in the semen sample (less than 1 million / ml).

Azoospermia is the absence of sperm in the semen.

Causes of Reduced Sperm Quality or Quantity

Certain lifestyle factors can impact the quality and quantity of sperm:

- Hot baths
- Tight underwear
- Smoking
- Alcohol
- Raised BMI
- Caffeine

Pre-Testicular Causes

Testosterone is necessary for sperm creation. The **hypothalamo-pituitary-gonadal axis** controls testosterone. **Hypogonadotrophic hypogonadism** (low **LH** and **FSH** resulting in low **testosterone**), can be due to:
- Pathology of the **pituitary gland** or **hypothalamus**
- Suppression due to stress, chronic conditions or hyperprolactinaemia
- Kallman syndrome

Testicular Causes

Testicular damage from:
- Mumps
- Undescended testes
- Trauma
- Radiotherapy
- Chemotherapy
- Cancer

Genetic or congenital disorders that result in defective or absent sperm production, such as:
- Klinefelter syndrome
- Y chromosome deletions
- Sertoli cell-only syndrome
- Anorchia (absent testes)

Post-Testicular Causes

Obstruction preventing sperm being ejaculated can be caused by:
- Damage to the testicle or vas deferens from trauma, surgery or cancer
- Ejaculatory duct obstruction
- Retrograde ejaculation
- Scarring from epididymitis, for example, caused by chlamydia
- Absence of the vas deferens (may be associated with cystic fibrosis)
- Young's syndrome (obstructive azoospermia, bronchiectasis and rhinosinusitis)

Investigations

The initial steps for investigating abnormal semen analysis include a history, examination, repeat sample and ultrasound of the testes.

Patients with abnormal semen results are referred to a urologist for further investigations. Further investigations that may be considered include:
- **Hormonal analysis** with **LH**, **FSH** and **testosterone** levels
- **Genetic testing**
- **Further imaging**, such as transrectal ultrasound or MRI
- **Vasography**, which involves injecting contrast into the vas deferens and performing xray to assess for obstruction
- **Testicular biopsy**

Management

Management depends on the underlying cause, and can involve:
- **Surgical sperm retrieval** where there is obstruction
- **Surgical correction** of an obstruction in the vas deferens
- **Intra-uterine insemination** involves separating high-quality sperm, then injecting them into the uterus
- **Intracytoplasmic sperm injection** (**ICSI**) involves injecting sperm directly into the cytoplasm of an egg
- **Donor insemination** involves sperm from a donor

In Vitro Fertilisation

In vitro fertilisation involves fertilising an egg with sperm in a lab, then injecting the resulting embryo into the uterus. There are many steps along the way, and it is a complicated and expensive process. As a result, funding criteria are very strict and vary between areas. Couples are limited to a set number of cycles funded by the NHS.

Each attempt has a roughly 25 - 30% success rate at producing a live birth.

Intrauterine insemination (**IUI**) is different from IVF. It is a more straightforward process, and involves injecting sperm into the uterus, avoiding intercourse. IUI is used in cases such as donor sperm for same-sex couples, HIV (avoiding unprotected sex) and practical issues with vaginal sex.

IVF Cycles

A cycle of IVF involves a single episode of **ovarian stimulation** and **collection of oocytes** (eggs). A single cycle may produce several **embryos**. Each of these embryos can be transferred separately in multiple attempts at pregnancy, all during one "cycle" of IVF. Embryos that are not used immediately may be frozen to be used at a later date. Frozen embryos can potentially be used years later, even after a successful pregnancy.

Process

There are a number of steps involved in the process of IVF:
- Suppressing the natural menstrual cycle
- Ovarian stimulation
- Oocyte collection
- Insemination or intracytoplasmic sperm injection (ICSI)
- Embryo culture
- Embryo transfer

Suppression of the Natural Menstrual Cycle

There are two protocols for the suppression of the natural menstrual cycle, preventing ovulation and ensuring the ovaries respond correctly to the **gonadotropins** (i.e. **FSH**). Suppression of the natural cycle involves either the use of **GnRH agonists** or **GnRH antagonists**. The choice between the **GnRH agonist** and **GnRH antagonist** protocol depends on individual factors.

For the **GnRH agonist protocol**, an injection of a **GnRH agonist** (e.g. **goserelin**) is given in the **luteal phase** of the menstrual cycle, around 7 days before the expected onset of the menstrual period (usually day 21 of the cycle). This initially stimulates the **pituitary gland** to secrete a large amount of **FSH** and **LH**. However, after this initial surge in FSH and LH, there is **negative feedback** to the **hypothalamus**, and the natural production of **GnRH** is **suppressed**. This causes suppression of the menstrual cycle.

For the **GnRH antagonist protocol**, daily **subcutaneous** injections of a **GnRH antagonist** (e.g. **cetrorelix**) are given, starting from day 5 - 6 of ovarian stimulation. This suppresses the body releasing LH and causing ovulation to occur.

Without suppression of the natural **gonadotropins** (**LH** and **FSH**) using one of the above protocols, ovulation would occur and the **follicles** that are developing would be released before it is possible to collect them.

Ovarian Stimulation

Ovarian stimulation involves using medications to promote the development of multiple **follicles** in the **ovaries**. This starts at the beginning of the menstrual cycle (usually day 2), with **subcutaneous** injections of **follicle-stimulating hormone** (**FSH**) over 10 to 14 days. The FSH stimulates the development of follicles, and this is closely monitored with regular transvaginal ultrasound scans.

When enough follicles have developed to an adequate size (usually around 18 millimetres), the FSH is stopped, and an injection of **human chorionic gonadotropin** (**hCG**) is given. This injection of HCG is given 36 hours before collection of the eggs. The hCG works similarly to what LH does naturally, and stimulates the final maturation of the follicles, ready for collection. This is referred to as a "**trigger injection**".

Oocyte Collection

The **oocytes** (eggs) are collected from the ovaries under the guidance of a transvaginal ultrasound scan. A needle is inserted through the vaginal wall into each ovary to aspirate the fluid from each **follicle**. This fluid contains the **mature oocytes** from the follicles. The procedure is usually performed under sedation (not a general anaesthetic). The fluid from the follicles is examined under the microscope for oocytes.

Oocyte Insemination

The male produces a semen sample around the time of oocyte collection. Frozen sperm from earlier samples may be used. The sperm and egg are mixed in a culture medium. Thousands of sperm need to be combined with each oocyte to produce enough enzymes (e.g. **hyaluronic acid**) for one sperm to penetrate the **corona radiata** and **zona pellucida** and fertilise the egg.

Intracytoplasmic Sperm Injection

Intracytoplasmic sperm injection (**ICSI**) is a treatment used mainly for **male factor infertility**, where there are a reduced number or quality of sperm. It is an addition to the IVF process. After the eggs are harvested, and a semen sample is produced, the highest quality sperm are isolated and injected directly into the cytoplasm of the egg.

Embryo Culture

Dishes containing the fertilised eggs are left in an incubator and observed over 2 - 5 days to see which will develop and grow. They are monitored until they reach the **blastocyst** stage of development (around day 5).

Embryo Transfer

After 2 - 5 days, the highest quality embryos are selected for transfer. A catheter is inserted under ultrasound guidance through the cervix into the uterus. A single embryo is injected through the catheter into the uterus, and the catheter is removed. Generally, only a single embryo is transferred. Two embryos may be transferred in older women (i.e. over 35 years). Any remaining embryos can be frozen for future attempts at transfer.

Pregnancy

A **pregnancy test** is performed around day 16 after egg collection. When this is positive, implantation has occurred. Even after a positive test, there is still the possibility of **miscarriage** or **ectopic** pregnancy.

When the pregnancy test is negative, implantation has failed. At this point, hormonal treatment is stopped. The woman will go on to have a menstrual period. The bleeding may be more substantial than usual given the additional hormones used during ovarian stimulation.

Progesterone is used from the time of oocyte collection until 8 - 10 weeks gestation, usually in the form of **vaginal suppositories**. This is to mimic the progesterone that would be released by the **corpus luteum** during a typical pregnancy. From 8 - 10 weeks the **placenta** takes over production of progesterone, and the suppositories are stopped.

An **ultrasound scan** is performed early in the pregnancy (around 7 weeks) to check for a fetal heartbeat, and rule out miscarriage or ectopic pregnancy. When the ultrasound scan confirms a healthy pregnancy, the remainder of the pregnancy can proceed with standard care, as with any other pregnancy.

Complications

The main complications relating to the overall process are:

- Failure
- Multiple pregnancy
- Ectopic pregnancy
- Ovarian hyperstimulation syndrome

There is a small risk of complications relating to the egg collection procedure:

- Pain
- Bleeding
- Pelvic infection
- Damage to the bladder or bowel

Ovarian Hyperstimulation Syndrome

Ovarian hyperstimulation syndrome (**OHSS**) is a complication of ovarian stimulation during IVF infertility treatment. It is associated with the use of **human chorionic gonadotropin** (**hCG**) to mature the follicles during the final steps of ovarian stimulation.

Pathophysiology

The primary mechanism for OHSS is an increase in **vascular endothelial growth factor** (**VEGF**) released by the **granulosa cells** of the **follicles**. VEGF increases **vascular permeability**, causing fluid to leak from capillaries. Fluid moves from the **intravascular space** to the **extravascular space**. This results in **oedema**, **ascites** and **hypovolaemia**.

The use of **gonadotrophins** (LH and FSH) during **ovarian stimulation** results in the development of multiple **follicles**. OHSS is provoked by the "**trigger injection**" of **hCG** 36 hours before **oocyte collection**. HCG stimulates the release of **VEGF** from the follicles. The features of the condition begin to develop after the hCG injection.

There is also activation of the **renin-angiotensin system**. A notable finding in patients with OOH is a **raised renin level**. The renin level correlates with the severity of the condition.

Risk Factors

- Younger age
- Lower BMI
- Raised anti-Müllerian hormone
- Higher antral follicle count
- Polycystic ovarian syndrome
- Raised oestrogen levels during ovarian stimulation

Prevention

Women are individually assessed for their risk of developing OHSS.

During stimulation with gonadotrophins, they are monitored with:
- **Serum oestrogen** levels (higher levels indicate a higher risk)
- **Ultrasound** monitoring of the follicles (higher number and larger size indicate a higher risk)

In women at higher risk, several strategies may be used to reduce the risk:
- Use of the GnRH antagonist protocol (rather than the GnRH agonist protocol)
- Lower doses of gonadotrophins
- Lower dose of the hCG injection
- Alternatives to the hCG injection (i.e. a GnRH agonist or LH)

Features

Early OHSS presents within 7 days of the hCG injection. Late OHSS presents from 10 days onwards.

Features of the condition include:
- Abdominal pain and bloating
- Nausea and vomiting
- Diarrhoea
- Hypotension
- Hypovolaemia
- Ascites
- Pleural effusions
- Renal failure
- Peritonitis from rupturing follicles releasing blood
- Prothrombotic state (risk of DVT and PE)

Severity

The severity is determined based on the clinical features:
- **Mild**: Abdominal pain and bloating
- **Moderate**: Nausea and vomiting with ascites seen on ultrasound
- **Severe**: Ascites, low urine output (*oliguria*), low serum albumin, high potassium and raised haematocrit (>45%)
- **Critical**: Tense ascites, no urine output (*anuria*), thromboembolism and acute respiratory distress syndrome (ARDS)

Management

Management is supportive with treatment of any complications. This involves:
- Oral fluids
- Monitoring urine output
- Low molecular weight heparin (to prevent thromboembolism)
- Ascitic fluid removal (*paracentesis*) if required
- IV colloids (e.g. human albumin solution)

Patients with mild to moderate OHSS are often managed as an outpatient. Severe cases require admission, and critical cases may require admission to the **intensive care unit** (**ICU**).

TOM TIP: Haematocrit may be monitored to assess the volume of fluid in the intravascular space. Haematocrit is the concentration of red blood cells in the blood. When the haematocrit goes up, this indicates less fluid in the intravascular space, as the blood is becoming more concentrated. Raised haematocrit can indicate dehydration.

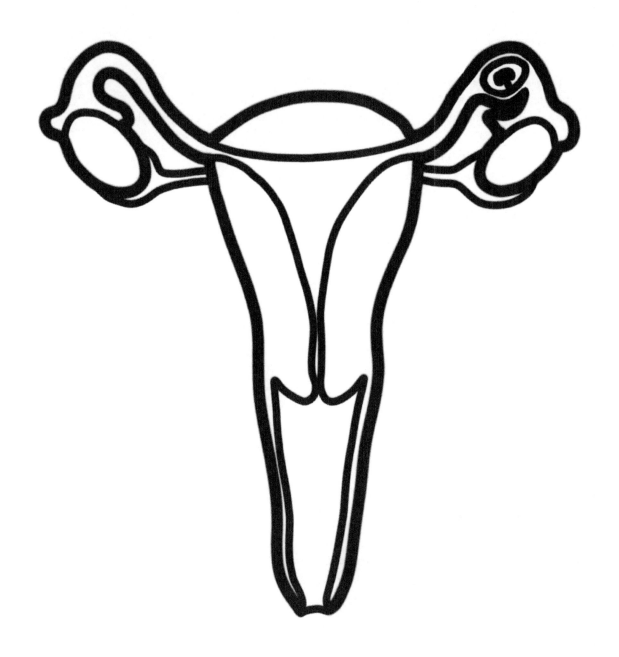

EARLY PREGNANCY

7.1	Ectopic Pregnancy	135
7.2	Miscarriage	138
7.3	Recurrent Miscarriage	140
7.4	Termination of Pregnancy	142
7.5	Nausea and Vomiting of Pregnancy	144
7.6	Molar Pregnancy	145

Ectopic Pregnancy

Ectopic pregnancy is when a pregnancy is implanted outside the uterus. The most common site is a **fallopian tube**. An ectopic pregnancy can also implant in the entrance to the fallopian tube (**cornual region**), ovary, cervix or abdomen.

Risk Factors

Certain factors can increase the risk of ectopic pregnancy:
- Previous ectopic pregnancy
- Previous pelvic inflammatory disease
- Previous surgery to the fallopian tubes
- Intrauterine devices (coils)
- Older age
- Smoking

Presentation

Ectopic pregnancy typically presents around 6 - 8 weeks gestation.

Have a low threshold for suspecting an ectopic pregnancy, even in atypical presentations. Always ask about the possibility of pregnancy, missed periods and recent unprotected sex in women presenting with lower abdominal pain.

The classic features of an ectopic pregnancy include:
- Missed period
- Constant lower abdominal pain in the right or left iliac fossa
- Vaginal bleeding
- Lower abdominal or pelvic tenderness
- Cervical motion tenderness (pain when moving the cervix during a bimanual examination)

It is also worth asking about:
- Dizziness or syncope (blood loss)
- Shoulder tip pain (peritonitis)

Ultrasound Findings

A **transvaginal ultrasound scan** is the investigation of choice for diagnosing an ectopic pregnancy. A **gestational sac** containing a **yolk sac** or **fetal pole** may be seen in a fallopian tube.

Sometimes a non-specific mass may be seen in the tube. When a mass containing an empty gestational sac is seen, this may be referred to as the "**blob sign**", "**bagel sign**" or "**tubal ring sign**" (all referring to the same appearance).

A mass representing a **tubal ectopic pregnancy** moves **separately** to the ovary. The mass may look similar to a **corpus luteum**; however, a corpus luteum will move **with** the ovary.

Features that may also indicate an ectopic pregnancy are:
- An empty uterus
- Fluid in the uterus, which may be mistaken as a gestational sac ("**pseudogestational** sac")

Pregnancy of Unknown Location

A *pregnancy of unknown location* (*PUL*) is when the woman has a positive pregnancy test and there is no evidence of pregnancy on the ultrasound scan. In this scenario, an ectopic pregnancy cannot be excluded, and careful follow up needs to be in place until a diagnosis can be confirmed.

Serum *human chorionic gonadotropin* (*hCG*) can be tracked over time to help monitor a pregnancy of unknown location. The serum hGC level is repeated after **48 hours**, to measure the change from baseline.

The developing **syncytiotrophoblast** of the pregnancy produces **hCG**. In an *intrauterine pregnancy*, the hCG will roughly **double every 48 hours**. This will not be the case in a *miscarriage* or *ectopic pregnancy*.

A **rise** of **more than 63%** after 48 hours is likely to indicate an *intrauterine pregnancy*. A repeat ultrasound scan is required after 1 - 2 weeks to confirm an intrauterine pregnancy. A pregnancy should be visible on an ultrasound scan once the hCG level is **above 1500** IU / l.

A **rise** of **less than 63%** after 48 hours may indicate an ectopic pregnancy. When this happens the patient needs close monitoring and review.

A **fall** of **more than 50%** is likely to indicate a miscarriage. A *urine pregnancy test* should be performed after 2 weeks to confirm the miscarriage is complete.

Monitoring the clinical signs and symptoms is more important than tracking the hCG level, and any change in symptoms needs careful assessment.

Management

Perform a pregnancy test in all women with abdominal or pelvic pain that may be caused by an ectopic pregnancy. Women with pelvic pain or tenderness and a positive pregnancy test need to be referred to an **early pregnancy assessment unit** (**EPAU**) or gynaecology service.

All ectopic pregnancies need to be terminated. An ectopic pregnancy is not a viable pregnancy.

There are three options for terminating an ectopic pregnancy:
- **Expectant management** (awaiting natural termination)
- **Medical management** (**methotrexate**)
- **Surgical management** (**salpingectomy** or **salpingotomy**)

Criteria for expectant management:
- Follow up needs to be possible to ensure successful termination
- The ectopic needs to be unruptured
- Adnexal mass < 35mm
- No visible heartbeat
- No significant pain
- HCG level < 1500 IU / l

Women with expectant management need careful follow up with close monitoring of hCG levels, and quick and easy access to services if their condition changes.

Criteria for **methotrexate** are the same as expectant management, except:
- HCG level must be < 5000 IU / l
- Confirmed absence of intrauterine pregnancy on ultrasound

Management with Methotrexate

Methotrexate is highly **teratogenic** (harmful to pregnancy). It is given as an **intramuscular injection** into a buttock. This halts the progress of the pregnancy and results in spontaneous termination.

Women treated with methotrexate are advised not to get pregnant for **3 months** following treatment. This is because the harmful effects of methotrexate on pregnancy can last this long.

Common side effects of methotrexate include:
- Vaginal bleeding
- Nausea and vomiting
- Abdominal pain
- Stomatitis (inflammation of the mouth)

Surgical Management

Anyone that does not meet the criteria for expectant or medical management requires surgical management. Most patients with an ectopic pregnancy will require surgical management. This include those with:
- Pain
- Adnexal mass > 35mm
- Visible heartbeat
- HCG levels > 5000 IU / l

There are two options for surgical management of ectopic pregnancy:
- **Laparoscopic salpingectomy**
- **Laparoscopic salpingotomy**

Laparoscopic salpingectomy is the first-line treatment for ectopic pregnancy. This involves a general anaesthetic and key-hole surgery with removal of the affected fallopian tube, along with the ectopic pregnancy inside the tube.

Laparoscopic salpingotomy may be used in women at increased risk of infertility due to damage to the other tube. The aim is to avoid removing the affected fallopian tube. A cut is made in the fallopian tube, the ectopic pregnancy is removed, and the tube is closed.

There is an increased risk of failure to remove the ectopic pregnancy with **salpingotomy** compared with **salpingectomy**. NICE state up to 1 in 5 women having **salpingotomy** may need further treatment with methotrexate or salpingectomy.

Anti-rhesus D prophylaxis is given to **rhesus negative** women having surgical management of ectopic pregnancy.

Miscarriage

Miscarriage is the spontaneous termination of a pregnancy. **Early miscarriage** is before 12 weeks gestation. **Late miscarriage** is between 12 and 24 weeks gestation.

Definitions

There are several definitions to remember relating to miscarriage:
- **Missed miscarriage** - the fetus is no longer alive, but no symptoms have occurred
- **Threatened miscarriage** - vaginal bleeding with a closed cervix and a fetus that is alive
- **Inevitable miscarriage** - vaginal bleeding with an open cervix
- **Incomplete miscarriage** - **retained products of conception** remain in the uterus after the miscarriage
- **Complete miscarriage** - a full miscarriage has occurred, and there are no products of conception left in the uterus
- **Anembryonic pregnancy** - a gestational sac is present but contains no embryo

Ultrasound Findings

A **transvaginal ultrasound scan** is the investigation of choice for diagnosing a miscarriage.

There are NICE guidelines (2019) and local protocols for diagnosing a miscarriage on ultrasound. Always check local and national guidelines when managing patients.

There are three key features that the sonographer looks for in an early pregnancy. These appear sequentially as the pregnancy develops. As each appears, the previous feature becomes less relevant in assessing the viability of the pregnancy. These features are:
- **Mean gestational sac diameter**
- **Fetal pole and crown-rump length**
- **Fetal heartbeat**

When a **fetal heartbeat** is visible, the pregnancy is considered **viable**. A **fetal heartbeat** is expected once the **crown-rump length** is **7mm** or more.

When the **crown-rump length** is less than **7mm**, **without** a fetal heartbeat, the scan is repeated after **at least** one week to ensure a heartbeat develops. When there is a **crown-rump length** of **7mm** or more, **without** a **fetal heartbeat**, the scan is repeated after one week before confirming a **non-viable pregnancy**.

A **fetal pole** is expected once the **mean gestational sac diameter** is **25mm** or more. When there is a **mean gestational sac diameter** of **25mm** or more, **without** a **fetal pole**, the scan is repeated after one week before confirming an **anembryonic pregnancy**.

Management

Less Than 6 Weeks Gestation
Women with a pregnancy **less than** 6 weeks' gestation presenting with bleeding can be managed **expectantly** provided they have no pain and no other complications or risk factors (e.g. previous ectopic). **Expectant management** before 6 weeks gestation involves awaiting the miscarriage without investigations or treatment. An ultrasound is unlikely to be helpful this early as the pregnancy will be too small to be seen.

A repeat urine pregnancy test is performed after 7 - 10 days, and if negative, a miscarriage can be confirmed. When bleeding continues, or pain occurs, referral and further investigation is indicated.

More Than 6 Weeks Gestation

The NICE guidelines (2019) suggest referral to an **early pregnancy assessment service** (**EPAU**) for women with a positive pregnancy test (more than 6 weeks gestation) and bleeding.

The early pregnancy assessment unit will arrange an **ultrasound scan**. Ultrasound will confirm the **location** and **viability** of the pregnancy. It is essential always to consider and exclude an **ectopic pregnancy**.

There are three options for managing a miscarriage:
- **Expectant management** (do nothing and await a spontaneous miscarriage)
- **Medical management** (misoprostol)
- **Surgical management**

Expectant Management

Expectant management is offered first-line for women without risk factors for heavy bleeding or infection. 1 - 2 weeks are given to allow the miscarriage to occur spontaneously. A repeat urine pregnancy test should be performed three weeks after bleeding and pain settle to confirm the miscarriage is complete.

Persistent or worsening bleeding requires further assessment and repeat ultrasound, as this may indicate an incomplete miscarriage and require additional management.

Medical Management

Misoprostol is a **prostaglandin analogue**, meaning it binds to **prostaglandin receptors** and activates them. Prostaglandins soften the cervix and stimulate uterine contractions.

Medical management of miscarriage involves using a dose of **misoprostol** to expedite the process of miscarriage. This can be as a **vaginal suppository** or an **oral** dose.

The key side effects of misoprostol are:
- Heavier bleeding
- Pain
- Vomiting
- Diarrhoea

Surgical Management

Surgical management can be performed under local or general anaesthetic.

There are two options for surgical management of a miscarriage:
- **Manual vacuum aspiration** under local anaesthetic as an outpatient
- **Electric vacuum aspiration** under general anaesthetic

Prostaglandins (**misoprostol**) are given before surgical management to soften the cervix.

Manual vacuum aspiration involves a **local anaesthetic** applied to the cervix. A tube attached to a specially designed syringe is inserted through the cervix into the uterus. The person performing the procedure then manually uses the syringe to aspirate contents of the uterus. To consider manual vacuum aspiration, women must find the process acceptable and be below 10 weeks gestation. It is more appropriate for women that have previously given birth (**parous** women).

Electric vacuum aspiration is the traditional surgical management of miscarriage. It involves a **general anaesthetic**. The operation is performed through the vagina and cervix without any incisions. The **cervix** is gradually widened using dilators, and the products of conception are removed through the cervix using an electric-powered vacuum.

Anti-rhesus D prophylaxis is given to **rhesus negative** women having surgical management of ectopic pregnancy.

Incomplete Miscarriage

An incomplete miscarriage occurs when **retained products of conception** (fetal or placental tissue) remain in the uterus after the miscarriage. Retained products create a risk of **infection**.

There are two options for treating an incomplete miscarriage:
- Medical management (**misoprostol**)
- Surgical management (**evacuation of retained products of conception**)

Evacuation of retained products of conception (**ERPC**) is a surgical procedure involving a **general anaesthetic**. The **cervix** is gradually widened using dilators, and the retained products are manually removed through the cervix using **vacuum aspiration** and **curettage** (scraping). A key complication is **endometritis** (infection of the endometrium) following the procedure.

Recurrent Miscarriage

Miscarriage is relatively common. Recurrent miscarriage is classed as **three or more consecutive** miscarriages.

The risk of miscarriage increases with age, with the rate of miscarriage approximately:
- 10% in women aged 20 - 30 years
- 15% in women aged 30 - 35 years
- 25% in women aged 35 - 45 years
- 50% in women aged 40 - 45 years

Investigations are initiated after:
- Three or more first-trimester miscarriages
- One or more second-trimester miscarriages

Causes

- **Idiopathic** (particularly in older women)
- **Antiphospholipid syndrome**
- **Hereditary thrombophilias**
- **Uterine abnormalities**
- **Genetic factors** in parents (e.g. **balanced translocations** in parental chromosomes)
- **Chronic histiocytic intervillositis**
- Other chronic diseases such as **diabetes**, untreated **thyroid disease** and **systemic lupus erythematosus** (**SLE**)

Antiphospholipid Syndrome

Antiphospholipid syndrome is a disorder associated with **antiphospholipid antibodies**, where blood becomes prone to clotting. The patient is in a **hyper-coagulable state**. The main associations are with **thrombosis** and complications in **pregnancy**, particularly **recurrent miscarriage**.

Antiphospholipid syndrome can occur on its own, or secondary to an autoimmune condition such as **systemic lupus erythematosus**.

The risk of miscarriage in patients with antiphospholipid syndrome is reduced by using both:
- Low dose aspirin
- Low molecular weight heparin (LMWH)

TOM TIP: If you remember one cause of recurrent miscarriages, remember antiphospholipid syndrome. Consider this in patients presenting in exams with recurrent miscarriages. There may be a past history of deep vein thrombosis. Test for antiphospholipid antibodies. Treatment is with aspirin and LMWH.

Hereditary Thrombophilias

The key inherited thrombophilias to remember are:
- Factor V Leiden (most common)
- Factor II (prothrombin) gene mutation
- Protein S deficiency

Uterine Abnormalities

Several uterine abnormalities can cause recurrent miscarriages:
- **Uterine septum** (a partition through the uterus)
- **Unicornuate uterus** (single-horned uterus)
- **Bicornuate uterus** (heart-shaped uterus)
- **Didelphic uterus** (double uterus)
- **Cervical insufficiency**
- **Fibroids**

Chronic Histiocytic Intervillositis

Chronic histiocytic intervillositis is a rare cause of recurrent miscarriage, particularly in the second trimester. It can also lead to intrauterine growth restriction (IUGR) and intrauterine death.

The condition is poorly understood. **Histiocytes** and **macrophages** build up in the placenta, causing inflammation and adverse outcomes. It is diagnosed by placental histology showing **infiltrates** of **mononuclear cells** in the **intervillous spaces**.

Investigations

Patients should be referred to a specialist in recurrent miscarriage for further investigation. Investigations include:
- Antiphospholipid antibodies
- Testing for hereditary thrombophilias
- Pelvic ultrasound
- Genetic testing of the **products of conception** from the third or future miscarriages
- Genetic testing on **parents**

Management

Management of recurrent miscarriage depends on the underlying cause.

There is new evidence from the **PRISM trial** that suggests a benefit to using **vaginal progesterone pessaries** during early pregnancy for women with **recurrent miscarriages** presenting with bleeding. This may become part of guidelines in the future. At present, the RCOG guidelines on recurrent miscarriage (2011) state there is insufficient evidence for progesterone supplementation.

Termination of Pregnancy

A termination of pregnancy (**TOP**), or **abortion**, involves an elective procedure to end a pregnancy.

Legal Requirements

The legal framework for a termination of pregnancy is the **1967 Abortion Act**. The **1990 Human Fertilisation and Embryology Act** altered and expanded the criteria for an abortion, and reduced the latest gestational age where an abortion is legal from 28 weeks to **24 weeks**.

There are specific criteria required to justify the decision to proceed with an abortion. The following is a simplified version of the criteria. An abortion can be performed before 24 weeks if *continuing* the pregnancy involves greater *risk* to the physical or mental health of:
- The woman
- Existing children of the family

The threshold for when the risk of continuing the pregnancy outweighs the risk of terminating the pregnancy is a matter of clinical judgement and opinion of the medical practitioners.

An abortion can be performed at any time during the pregnancy if:
- Continuing the pregnancy is likely to risk the life of the woman
- Terminating the pregnancy will prevent "grave permanent injury" to the physical or mental health of the woman
- There is "substantial risk" that the child would suffer physical or mental abnormalities making it seriously handicapped

The legal requirements for an abortion are:
- Two registered medical practitioners must sign to agree abortion is indicated
- It must be carried out by a registered medical practitioner in an NHS hospital or approved premise

Pre-Abortion Care

Abortion services can be accessed by self-referral or by GP, GUM or family planning clinic referral. Doctors who object to abortions should pass on to another doctor able to make the referral. Many abortion services are accessed by self-referral, without the involvement of a GP or other doctor to make the referral.

Marie Stopes UK is a charity that provides abortion services. They offer a remote service for women less than 10 weeks gestation, where consultations are held by telephone and medication are issued remotely to be taken at home.

Women should be offered counselling and information to help decision making from a trained practitioner. Informed consent is essential.

Medical Abortion

A medical abortion is most appropriate earlier in pregnancy, but can be used at any gestation. It involves two treatments:
- **Mifepristone** (anti-progestogen)
- **Misoprostol** (prostaglandin analogue), taken 1 - 2 days after mifepristone

Mifepristone is an **anti-progestogen** medication that blocks the action of **progesterone**, halting the pregnancy and relaxing the cervix.

Misoprostol is a **prostaglandin analogue**, meaning it binds to **prostaglandin receptors** and activates them. Prostaglandins soften the cervix and stimulate uterine contractions. From 10 weeks gestation, additional misoprostol doses (e.g. every 3 hours) are required until expulsion.

Rhesus negative women with a gestational age of **10 weeks or above** having a medical TOP should have anti-D prophylaxis.

Surgical Abortion

Surgical abortion can be performed, depending on preference and gestational age, under:
- Local anaesthetic
- Local anaesthetic plus sedation
- General anaesthetic

Prior to surgical abortion, medications are used for **cervical priming**. This involves softening and dilating the cervix with **misoprostol**, **mifepristone** or **osmotic dilators**. Osmotic dilators are devices inserted into the cervix, that gradually expand as they absorb fluid, opening the cervical canal.

There are two options for surgical abortion:
- Cervical dilatation and suction of the contents of the uterus (usually up to 14 weeks)
- Cervical dilatation and evacuation using forceps (between 14 and 24 weeks)

Rhesus negative women having a surgical TOP should have anti-D prophylaxis. The NICE guidelines (2019) say it should be *considered* in women less than 10 weeks gestation.

Post-Abortion Care

Women may experience vaginal bleeding and abdominal cramps intermittently for up to 2 weeks after the procedure. A urine pregnancy test is performed 3 weeks after the abortion to confirm it is complete. Contraception is discussed and started where appropriate. Support and counselling is offered.

Complications

- Bleeding
- Pain
- Infection
- Failure of the abortion (pregnancy continues)
- Damage to the cervix, uterus or other structures

Nausea and Vomiting of Pregnancy

Nausea is a common symptom in pregnancy, particularly early on. Nausea and vomiting in pregnancy starts in the first trimester, peaking around 8 - 12 weeks gestation. The severe form of nausea and vomiting in pregnancy is called **hyperemesis gravidarum**. **Hyper-** refers to lots, **-emesis** refers to vomiting and **gravida-** relates to pregnancy.

Nausea and vomiting are normal during early pregnancy. Symptoms usually start from 4 - 7 weeks, are worst around 10 - 12 weeks and resolve by 16 - 20 weeks. Symptoms can persist throughout pregnancy.

The **placenta** produces **human chorionic gonadotropin** (**hCG**) during pregnancy. This hormone is thought to be responsible for nausea and vomiting. Theoretically, higher levels of hCG result in worse symptoms.

Nausea and vomiting are more severe in **molar pregnancies** and **multiple pregnancies** due to the higher hCG levels. It also tends to be worse in the first pregnancy, and overweight or obese women.

Diagnosis

Nausea and vomiting of pregnancy can be diagnosed based on a typical history. Nausea and vomiting needs to start in the first trimester, and other causes need to be excluded before making a diagnosis.

Hyperemesis Gravidarum

Hyperemesis gravidarum is the severe form of nausea and vomiting in pregnancy. The RCOG guideline (2016) criteria for diagnosing hyperemesis gravidarum are "**protracted**" nausea and vomiting, plus:
- More than 5 % weight loss compared with before pregnancy
- Dehydration
- Electrolyte imbalance

Assessing the Severity

The severity can be assessed using the **Pregnancy-Unique Quantification of Emesis** (**PUQE**) score. This gives a score out of 15:
- Less than 7: Mild
- 7 - 12: Moderate
- More than 12: Severe

Management

Antiemetics are used to suppress nausea. Vaguely in order of preference and known safety, the choices are:
1. Prochlorperazine (stemetil)
2. Cyclizine
3. Ondansetron
4. Metoclopramide

Ranitidine or **omeprazole** can be used if acid reflux is a problem.

The RCOG also suggest complementary therapies that may be considered by the woman:
- Ginger
- Acupressure on the wrist at the PC6 point (inner wrist) may improve symptoms

Mild cases can be managed with oral antiemetics at home. **Admission** should be considered when:
- Unable to tolerate oral antiemetics or keep down any fluids
- More than 5 % weight loss compared with pre-pregnancy
- **Ketones** are present in the urine on a urine dipstick (2 + ketones on the urine dipstick is significant)
- Other medical conditions need treating that required admission

Moderate-severe cases may require **ambulatory care** (e.g. early pregnancy assessment unit) or **admission** for:
- IV or IM antiemetics
- IV fluids (normal saline with added potassium chloride)
- Daily monitoring of U&Es while having IV therapy
- **Thiamine supplementation** to prevent deficiency (prevents **Wernicke-Korsakoff syndrome**)
- **Thromboprophylaxis** (TED stocking and low molecular weight heparin) during admission

Molar Pregnancy

An **hydatiform mole** is a type of tumour that grows like a pregnancy inside the uterus. This is called a **molar pregnancy**. There are two types of molar pregnancy: a **complete mole** and a **partial mole**.

A **complete mole** occurs when two sperm cells fertilise an ovum that contains no genetic material (an "empty ovum"). These sperm then combine genetic material, and the cells start to divide and grow into a tumour called a **complete mole**. No fetal material will form.

A **partial mole** occurs when two sperm cells fertilise a normal ovum (containing genetic material) at the same time. The new cell now has three sets of chromosomes. The cell divides and multiplies into a tumour called a **partial mole**. In a partial mole, some fetal material may form.

Diagnosis

Molar pregnancy behaves like a normal pregnancy. Periods will stop and the hormonal changes of pregnancy will occur. There are a few things that can indicate a molar pregnancy versus a normal pregnancy:
- More severe morning sickness
- Vaginal bleeding
- Increased enlargement of the uterus
- Abnormally high hCG
- Thyrotoxicosis (hCG can mimic TSH and stimulate the thyroid to produce excess T3 and T4)

Ultrasound of the pelvis shows a characteristic "**snowstorm appearance**" of the pregnancy.

A provisional diagnosis can be made by **ultrasound** and confirmed with **histology** of the mole after evacuation.

Management

Management involves **evacuation of the uterus** to remove the mole. The products of conception need to be sent for **histological examination** to confirm a molar pregnancy. Patients should be referred to the **gestational trophoblastic disease centre** for management and follow up. The **hCG levels** are monitored until they return to normal. Occasionally the mole can **metastasise**, and the patient may require **systemic chemotherapy**.

ANTENATAL CARE

8.1	Pregnancy Timeline	147
8.2	Pregnancy Lifestyle Advice	148
8.3	Booking Clinic	150
8.4	Antenatal Screening for Down's Syndrome	151
8.5	Chronic Conditions in Pregnancy	152
8.6	Medications and Pregnancy	153
8.7	Infections in Pregnancy	155
8.8	Rhesus Incompatibility	158
8.9	Small for Gestational Age	159
8.10	Large for Gestational Age	162
8.11	Multiple Pregnancy	163
8.12	Urinary Tract Infection in Pregnancy	165
8.13	Anaemia in Pregnancy	166
8.14	Venous Thromboembolism in Pregnancy	168
8.15	Pre-eclampsia	171
8.16	Gestational Diabetes	174
8.17	Obstetric Cholestasis	176
8.18	Acute Fatty Liver of Pregnancy	178
8.19	Pregnancy-Related Rashes	179
8.20	Placenta Praevia	181
8.21	Vasa Praevia	182
8.22	Placental Abruption	183
8.23	Placenta Accreta	185
8.24	Breech Presentation	186
8.25	Stillbirth	187
8.26	Cardiac Arrest in Pregnancy	189

Pregnancy Timeline

There are several key definitions to become familiar with:
- **Last menstrual period** (**LMP**) refers to the date of the first day of the most recent menstrual period
- **Gestational age** (**GA**) refers to the duration of the pregnancy starting from the date of the *last menstrual period*
- **Estimated date of delivery** (**EDD**) refers to the estimated date of delivery (40 weeks gestation)
- **Gravida** (**G**) is the total number of pregnancies a woman has had
- **Primigravida** refers to a patient that is pregnant for the first time
- **Multigravida** refers to a patient that is pregnant for at least the second time
- **Para** (**P**) refers to the number of times the woman has given birth after 24 weeks gestation, regardless of whether the fetus was alive or stillborn
- **Nulliparous** ("**nullip**") refers to a patient that has never given birth after 24 weeks gestation
- **Primiparous** technically refers to a patient that has given birth after 24 weeks gestation once before (see below)
- **Multiparous** ("**multip**") refers to a patient that has given birth after 24 weeks gestation two or more times

TOM TIP: The term primiparous, or "primip" is a bit confusing. Technically, it refers to a woman that has given birth once before. However, it is often used on the labour ward to refer to a woman that is due to give birth for the first time (and has never given birth before). You may hear patients referred to on the labour ward as a "primip" when they have never given birth before.

The timeline for each pregnancy depends on the start date of the **last menstrual period** (**LMP**). This determines the **gestational age** (**GA**) and the **estimated date of delivery** (**EDD**) of the pregnancy. After the booking scan, the **gestational age** is more accurately assessed and the **estimated date of delivery** is updated accordingly.

The gestational age is described in weeks and days. For example:
- **5 + 0** refers to 5 weeks gestational age (since the LMP)
- **13 + 6** refers to 13 weeks and 6 days gestational age

Gravidity and Parity

It is worth becoming familiar with **gravida** (**G**) and **para** (**P**), as you will find this written on medical records. Here are some examples:
- A pregnant woman with three previous deliveries at term: **G4 P3**
- A non-pregnant woman with a previous birth of healthy **twins**: **G1 P1**
- A non-pregnant woman with a previous **miscarriage**: **G1 P0 + 1**
- A non-pregnant woman with a previous **stillbirth** (after 24 weeks gestation): **G1 P1**

Trimesters

The **first trimester** is from the start of pregnancy until 12 weeks gestation.

The **second trimester** is from 13 weeks until 26 weeks gestation.

The **third trimester** is from 27 weeks gestation until birth.

It is worth noting that **fetal movements** start from around 20 weeks gestation, and continue until birth.

Key Milestones

Dates	Event	Purpose
Before 10 weeks	Booking clinic	Offer a baseline assessment and plan the pregnancy
Between 10 and 13 + 6	Dating scan	An accurate **gestational age** is calculated from the **crown rump length** (**CRL**), and multiple pregnancies are identified
16 weeks	Antenatal appointment	Discuss results and plan future appointments
Between 18 and 20 + 6	Anomaly scan	An ultrasound to identify any anomalies, such as heart conditions
25, 28, 31, 34, 36, 38, 40, 41 and 42 weeks	Antenatal appointments	Monitor the pregnancy and discuss future plans

Additional Milestones

There may be additional appointments necessary if the woman fits certain criteria:
- **Additional appointments** for higher risk or complicated pregnancies
- **Oral glucose tolerance test** in women at risk of **gestational diabetes** (between 24 - 28 weeks)
- **Anti-D injections** in **rhesus negative** women (at 28 and 34 weeks)
- **Ultrasound scan** at 32 weeks for women with **placenta praevia** on the anomaly scan
- **Serial growth scans** are offered to women at increased risk of **fetal growth restriction**

Routine Antenatal Appointments

Several things are covered at each routine antenatal appointment:
- Discuss plans for the remainder of the pregnancy and delivery
- **Symphysis–fundal height** measurement from 24 weeks onwards
- **Fetal presentation** assessment from 36 weeks onwards
- **Urine dipstick** for **protein** for pre-eclampsia
- **Blood pressure** for pre-eclampsia
- **Urine** for microscopy and culture for asymptomatic bacteriuria

Vaccines

There are two vaccines offered to all pregnant women:
- **Whooping cough** (**pertussis**) from 16 weeks gestation
- **Influenza** (**flu**) when available in autumn or winter

Live vaccines, such as the MMR vaccine, are avoided in pregnancy.

Pregnancy Lifestyle Advice

The general lifestyle advice for pregnant women includes:

- Take **folic acid** 400mcg from before pregnancy to 12 weeks (reduces neural tube defects)
- Take **vitamin D** supplement (10 mcg or 400 IU daily)
- Avoid **vitamin A** supplements and eating liver or pate (**vitamin A** is **teratogenic** at high doses)
- **Don't drink alcohol** when pregnant (risk of fetal alcohol syndrome)
- **Don't smoke** (smoking has a long list of complications, see below)
- Avoid unpasteurised dairy or blue cheese (risk of **listeriosis**)
- Avoid undercooked or raw poultry (risk of **salmonella**)
- Continue moderate exercise but avoid **contact sports**
- Sex is safe
- Flying increases the risk of **venous thromboembolism** (VTE)
- Place car seatbelts above and below the bump (not across it)

Alcohol

Alcohol can cross the placenta, enter the fetus, and disrupt fetal development. There is no safe level of alcohol in pregnancy. Pregnant women are encouraged not to drink alcohol at all. Small amounts are less likely to result in lasting effects. The effects are greatest in the first 3 months of pregnancy.

Alcohol in early pregnancy can lead to:
- Miscarriage
- Small for dates
- Preterm delivery
- Fetal alcohol syndrome

Fetal alcohol syndrome refers to certain characteristics that can occur in children of mothers that consumed alcohol during pregnancy. The features include:
- **Microcephaly** (small head)
- **Thin upper lip**
- **Smooth flat philtrum** (the groove between the nose and upper lip)
- **Short palpebral fissure** (short horizontal distance from one side of the eye to the other)
- **Learning disability**
- **Behavioural difficulties**
- **Hearing** and **vision problems**
- **Cerebral palsy**

Smoking in pregnancy

Smoking in pregnancy increases the risk of:
- **Fetal growth restriction** (**FGR**)
- Miscarriage
- Stillbirth
- Preterm labour and delivery
- Placental abruption
- Pre-eclampsia
- Cleft lip or palate
- **Sudden infant death syndrome** (**SIDS**)

Flying in Pregnancy

The RCOG advises flying is generally ok in uncomplicated healthy pregnancies up to:
- 37 weeks in a single pregnancy
- 32 weeks in a twin pregnancy

After 28 weeks gestation, most airlines need a note from a midwife, GP or obstetrician to state the pregnancy is going well and there are no additional risks.

Booking Clinic

The booking clinic is the initial appointment to discuss and arrange plans for the pregnancy. This ideally occurs before 10 weeks gestation. The woman meets with a midwife to discuss all aspects of pregnancy. She will get a green book that documents the progress during the pregnancy.

Education

Pregnancy-related topics are covered during the booking clinic:
- What to expect at different stages of pregnancy
- Lifestyle advice in pregnancy (e.g. not smoking)
- Supplements (e.g. folic acid and vitamin D)
- Plans for birth
- Screening tests (e.g. Downs screening)
- Antenatal classes
- Breastfeeding classes
- Discuss mental health

Booking Bloods

A set of **booking bloods** are taken for:
- Blood group, antibodies and rhesus D status
- Full blood count for anaemia
- Screening for **thalassaemia** (all women) and **sickle cell disease** (women at higher risk)

Patients are also offered screening for infectious diseases, by testing antibodies for:
- HIV
- Hepatitis B
- Syphilis

Screening for Down's syndrome may be initiated depending on the gestational age. Bloods required for the **combined test** are taken from 11 weeks onwards.

Other Measures

- Weight, height and BMI
- Urine for protein and bacteria
- Blood pressure
- Discuss female genital mutilation
- Discuss domestic violence

Risk Assessment

Women are assessed for risk factors for other conditions, and plans are put in place with additional appointments booked. These conditions include:
- **Rhesus negative** (book **anti-D prophylaxis**)
- **Gestational diabetes** (book **oral glucose tolerance test**)
- **Fetal growth restriction** (book additional **growth scans**)
- **Venous thromboembolism** (provide **prophylactic LMWH** if high risk)
- **Pre-eclampsia** (provide **aspirin** if high risk)

Antenatal Screening for Down's Syndrome

Down's syndrome is a condition caused by three copies of **chromosome 21**. It is also called **trisomy 21**. It gives characteristic **dysmorphic features** and has many associated conditions. The extent to which a person is affected and the related conditions they have vary between individuals.

All women are offered screening for Down's syndrome during pregnancy. The purpose of the screening test is to decide which women should receive more invasive tests to establish a definitive diagnosis.

It is the choice of the woman whether to go ahead with screening. The screening tests involve taking measurements from the fetus using ultrasound, combining those measurements with the mother's age and blood results and providing an indication of the risk of Down's syndrome. Older mothers have a higher risk of Down's syndrome.

Combined Test

The **combined test** is the first-line and the most accurate screening test. It is performed between 11 and 14 weeks gestation, and involves combining results from **ultrasound** and **maternal blood tests**.

Ultrasound measures **nuchal translucency**, which is the thickness of the back of the neck of the fetus. Down's syndrome is one cause of a nuchal thickness greater than 6mm.

Maternal blood tests:
- **Beta-human chorionic gonadotrophin (beta-hCG)** - a higher result indicates a greater risk
- **Pregnancy-associated plasma protein-A (PAPPA)** - a lower result indicates a greater risk

Triple Test

The **triple test** is performed between 14 and 20 weeks gestation. It only involves **maternal blood tests**:
- **Beta-hCG** - a **higher** result indicates greater risk
- **Alpha-fetoprotein (AFP)** - a **lower** result indicates a greater risk
- **Serum oestriol** (female sex hormone) - a **lower** result indicates a greater risk

Quadruple Test

The **quadruple test** is performed between 14 and 20 weeks gestation. It is identical to the triple test, but also includes maternal blood testing for **inhibin-A**. A **higher** inhibin-A indicates a greater risk.

Antenatal Testing for Down's Syndrome

The screening tests provide a **risk score** for the fetus having Down's syndrome. When the risk of Down's is greater than **1 in 150** (occurs in around 5% of tested women), the woman is offered **amniocentesis** or **chorionic villus sampling**.

These tests involve taking a sample of the fetal cells to perform **karyotyping** for a definitive answer about Down's:
- **Chorionic villus sampling (CVS)** involves an ultrasound-guided biopsy of the placental tissue. This is used when testing is done earlier in pregnancy (before 15 weeks).
- **Amniocentesis** involves ultrasound-guided aspiration of amniotic fluid using a needle and syringe. This is used later in pregnancy once there is enough amniotic fluid to make it safer to take a sample.

Non-Invasive Prenatal Testing

Non-invasive prenatal testing (**NIPT**) is a relatively new test for detecting abnormalities in the fetus during pregnancy. It involves a simple blood test from the mother. The blood will contain fragments of DNA, some of which will come from the placental tissue and represent the fetal DNA. These fragments can be analysed to detect conditions such as Down's.

NIPT is not a definitive test, but it does give a very good indication of whether the fetus is affected. NIPT is gradually being rolled out in the NHS as an alternative to invasive testing (CVS and amniocentesis) for women that have a higher than 1 in 150 risk of Down's syndrome.

Chronic Conditions in Pregnancy

Women with existing health conditions may need additional management of both the existing health condition and the pregnancy. They are generally managed jointly by the obstetric team and the specialist in their health condition.

Hypothyroidism in Pregnancy

Untreated or under-treated hypothyroidism in pregnancy can lead to several adverse pregnancy outcomes, including miscarriage, anaemia, small for gestational age and pre-eclampsia.

Hypothyroidism is treated with **levothyroxine** (T4). Levothyroxine can cross the **placenta** and provide thyroid hormone to the developing fetus. The levothyroxine dose needs to be **increased** during pregnancy, usually by at least 25 - 50 mcg (30 - 50%). Treatment is titrated based on the TSH level, aiming for a low-normal TSH level.

Hypertension

Women with existing hypertension may need changes to their medications.

Medications that should be stopped as they may cause congenital abnormalities:
- ACE inhibitors (e.g. ramipril)
- Angiotensin receptor blockers (e.g. losartan)
- Thiazide and thiazide-like diuretics (e.g. indapamide)

Medications that are not known to be harmful:
- Labetalol (a beta-blocker - although other beta-blockers may have adverse effects)
- Calcium channel blockers (e.g. nifedipine)
- Alpha-blockers (e.g. doxazosin)

Epilepsy in Pregnancy

Women with epilepsy should take folic acid 5mg daily from before conception to reduce the risk of **neural tube defects**.

Pregnancy may worsen seizure control due to the additional stress, lack of sleep, hormonal changes and altered medication regimes. Seizures are not known to be harmful to the pregnancy, other than the risk of physical injury.

Ideally, epilepsy should be controlled with a single anti-epileptic drug before becoming pregnant.

Regarding anti-epileptic drugs:
- **Levetiracetam**, **lamotrigine** and **carbamazepine** are the safer anti-epileptic medications in pregnancy
- **Sodium valproate** is **avoided** as it causes neural tube defects and developmental delay
- **Phenytoin** is **avoided** as it causes cleft lip and palate

There are a lot of warnings about the **teratogenic** effects of **sodium valproate**, and NICE updated their guidelines in 2018 to reflect this. It must be avoided in girls or women unless there are no suitable alternatives and strict criteria are met to ensure they do not get pregnant. There is a specific program called **Prevent** (**valproate pregnancy prevention programme**) to ensure this happens.

Rheumatoid Arthritis

Rheumatoid arthritis is an autoimmune condition that causes **chronic inflammation** of the **synovial lining** of the **joints**, **tendon sheaths** and **bursa**. It is an **inflammatory arthritis**. It is treated with **disease-modifying anti-rheumatic drugs** (**DMARDs**).

Ideally, rheumatoid arthritis should be well controlled for at least three months before becoming pregnant. Often the symptoms of rheumatoid arthritis will improve during pregnancy, and may flare up after delivery.

The treatment regime may need to be altered by a specialist rheumatologist before and during pregnancy:
- **Methotrexate** is contraindicated, and is teratogenic, causing miscarriage and congenital abnormalities
- **Hydroxychloroquine** is considered safe during pregnancy and is often the first-line choice
- **Sulfasalazine** is considered safe during pregnancy
- **Corticosteroids** may be used during flare-ups

Medications and Pregnancy

The effects of certain medications during pregnancy may be tested in exams, and they are worth being aware of when prescribing for women that are, or could be, pregnant. This is not an exhaustive list, and when in doubt always check the BNF, guidelines and with seniors when prescribing in pregnancy.

Non-Steroidal Anti-Inflammatory Drugs

Examples of non-steroidal anti-inflammatory drugs (**NSAIDs**) are **ibuprofen** and **naproxen**. They work by blocking **prostaglandins**. Prostaglandins are important in maintaining the **ductus arteriosus** in the fetus and neonate. Prostaglandins also soften the **cervix** and stimulate **uterine contractions** at the time of delivery.

NSAIDS are generally avoided in pregnancy unless really necessary (e.g. in rheumatoid arthritis). They are particularly avoided in the third trimester, as they can cause premature **closure of the ductus arteriosus** in the fetus. They can also **delay labour**.

Beta-Blockers

Beta-blockers are commonly used for hypertension, cardiac conditions and migraine. Labetalol is the most frequently used beta-blocker in pregnancy, and is first-line for high blood pressure caused by pre-eclampsia.

Beta-blockers can cause:
- Fetal growth restriction
- Hypoglycaemia in the neonate
- Bradycardia in the neonate

ACE Inhibitors and Angiotensin II Receptor Blockers

Medications that block the **renin-angiotensin system** (ACE inhibitors and ARBs) can cross the placenta and enter the fetus. In the fetus, they mainly affect the kidneys, and reduce the production of urine (and therefore amniotic fluid). The other notably effect is **hypocalvaria**, which is an incomplete formation of the skull bones.

ACE inhibitors and ARBs, when used in pregnancy, can cause:
- **Oligohydramnios** (reduced amniotic fluid)
- Miscarriage or fetal death
- **Hypocalvaria** (incomplete formation of the skull bones)
- Renal failure in the neonate
- Hypotension in the neonate

Opiates

The use of opiates during pregnancy can cause **withdrawal symptoms** in the neonate after birth. This is called **neonatal abstinence syndrome** (**NAS**). NAS presents between 3 – 72 hours after birth with irritability, tachypnoea (fast breathing), high temperatures and poor feeding.

Warfarin

Warfarin may be used in younger patients with recurrent venous thrombosis, atrial fibrillation or metallic mechanical heart valves. It crosses the placenta and is considered teratogenic in pregnancy, therefore it is avoided in pregnant women. Warfarin can cause:
- Fetal loss
- Congenital malformations, particularly craniofacial problems
- Bleeding during pregnancy, postpartum haemorrhage, fetal haemorrhage and intracranial bleeding

Sodium Valproate

The use of sodium valproate in pregnancy causes **neural tube defects** and **developmental delay**.

There are strict rules for avoiding sodium valproate in girls or women unless there are no suitable alternatives and strict criteria are met to ensure they do not get pregnant. There is a specific program called **Prevent** (**valproate pregnancy prevention programme**) to ensure this happens.

Lithium

Lithium is used as a mood stabilising medication for patients with bipolar disorder, mania and recurrent depression. It is avoided in pregnant women or those planning pregnancy unless other options (i.e. antipsychotics) have failed.

Lithium is particularly avoided in the first trimester, as it is linked with **congenital cardiac abnormalities**. In particular, it is associated with **Ebstein's anomaly**, where the tricuspid valve is set lower on the right side of the heart (towards the apex), causing a bigger right atrium and a smaller right ventricle.

When lithium is used, levels need to be monitored closely (NICE say every four weeks, then weekly from 36 weeks). Lithium also enters breast milk and is toxic to the infant, so should be avoided in breastfeeding.

Selective Serotonin Reuptake Inhibitors

Selective serotonin reuptake inhibitors (**SSRIs**) are the most commonly used antidepressants in pregnancy. SSRIs can cross the placenta into the fetus. The risks need to be balanced against the benefits of treatment. The risks associated with untreated depression can be very significant. Women need to be aware of the potential risks of SSRIs in pregnancy:
- **First-trimester** use has a link with **congenital heart defects**
- **First-trimester** use of **paroxetine** has a stronger link with **congenital malformations**
- **Third-trimester** use has a link with **persistent pulmonary hypertension** in the neonate
- **Neonates** can experience **withdrawal symptoms**, usually only mild and not requiring medical management

Isotretinoin (Roaccutane)

Isotretinoin is a **retinoid** medication (relating to **vitamin A**) that is used to treat **severe acne**. It should be prescribed and monitored by a specialist dermatologist.

Isotretinoin is highly teratogenic, causing miscarriage and congenital defects. Women need very reliable contraception before, during and for one month after taking isotretinoin.

Infections in Pregnancy

Rubella

Rubella is also known as **German measles**. **Congenital rubella syndrome** is caused by maternal infection with the **rubella virus** during the first **20 weeks** of pregnancy. The risk is highest before ten weeks gestation.

Women **planning** to become pregnant should ensure they have had the **MMR vaccine**. When in doubt, they can be tested for **rubella immunity**. If they do not have **antibodies** to **rubella**, they can be **vaccinated** with two doses of the MMR, three months apart.

Pregnant women **should not** receive the MMR vaccination, as this is a **live vaccine**. Non-immune women should be offered the vaccine **after** giving birth.

The features of congenital rubella syndrome to be aware of are:
- Congenital deafness
- Congenital cataracts
- Congenital heart disease (PDA and pulmonary stenosis)
- Learning disability

Chickenpox

Chickenpox is caused by the **varicella zoster virus** (**VZV**). It is dangerous in pregnancy because it can lead to:
- More severe cases in the mother, such as **varicella pneumonitis**, **hepatitis** or **encephalitis**
- Fetal varicella syndrome
- Severe **neonatal varicella infection** (if infected around delivery)

Mothers that have previously had chickenpox are immune and safe. When in doubt, **IgG** levels for **VZV** can be tested. A positive IgG for VZV indicates immunity. Women that are not immune to varicella may be offered the varicella vaccine before or after pregnancy.

Exposure to chickenpox in pregnancy:
- When the pregnant woman has previously had chickenpox, they are safe
- When they are not sure about their immunity, test the VZV IgG levels. If positive, they are safe.
- When they are not immune, they can be treated with **IV varicella immunoglobulins** as prophylaxis against developing chickenpox. This should be given within ten days of exposure.

When the chickenpox rash starts in pregnancy, they may be treated with oral aciclovir if they present within 24 hours and are more than 20 weeks gestation.

Congenital varicella syndrome occurs in around 1% of cases of chickenpox in pregnancy. It occurs when infection occurs in the first 28 weeks of gestation. The typical features include:
- Fetal growth restriction
- Microcephaly, hydrocephalus and learning disability
- Scars and significant skin changes located in specific **dermatomes**
- Limb **hypoplasia** (underdeveloped limbs)
- Cataracts and inflammation in the eye (**chorioretinitis**)

Listeria

Listeria is an infectious **gram-positive** bacteria that causes listeriosis. Listeriosis is many times more likely in pregnant women compared with non-pregnant individuals. Infection in the mother may be asymptomatic, cause a flu-like illness, or less commonly cause pneumonia or meningoencephalitis.

Listeriosis in pregnant women has a high rate of **miscarriage** or **fetal death**. It can also cause **severe neonatal infection**.

Listeria is typically transmitted by **unpasteurised dairy products**, **processed meats** and contaminated foods. Pregnant women are advised to avoid high-risk foods (e.g. **blue cheese**) and practice good food hygiene.

Congenital Cytomegalovirus

Congenital cytomegalovirus infection occurs due to a cytomegalovirus (CMV) infection in the mother during pregnancy. The virus is mostly spread via the infected saliva or urine of asymptomatic children. Most cases of CMV in pregnancy do not cause congenital CMV.

The features of **congenital CMV** are:
- Fetal growth restriction
- Microcephaly
- Hearing loss
- Vision loss
- Learning disability
- Seizures

Congenital Toxoplasmosis

Infection with the **Toxoplasma gondii** parasite is usually asymptomatic. It is primarily spread by contamination with faeces from a cat that is a **host** of the parasite. When infection occurs during pregnancy, it can lead to **congenital toxoplasmosis**. The risk is higher later in the pregnancy.

There is a **classic triad** of features in congenital toxoplasmosis:
- Intracranial calcification
- Hydrocephalus
- Chorioretinitis (inflammation of the choroid and retina in the eye)

Parvovirus B19

Parvovirus B19 infection typically affects children. It is also known as **fifth disease**, **slapped cheek syndrome** and **erythema infectiosum**. It is caused by the **parvovirus B19** virus. The illness is self-limiting, and the rash and symptoms usually fade over 1 – 2 weeks.

Parvovirus infection starts with non-specific viral symptoms. After 2 – 5 days, the rash appears quite rapidly as a diffuse bright red rash on both cheeks, as though they have "**slapped cheeks**". A few days later a **reticular** mildly erythematous rash affecting the trunk and limbs appears, which can be raised and itchy. Reticular means net-like.

Healthy children and adults have a low risk of complications, and management is supportive. They are infectious 7 - 10 days before the rash appears. They are not infectious once the rash has appeared. Significant exposure to parvovirus is classed as 15 minutes in the same room, or face-to-face contact, with someone that has the virus.

Infections with parvovirus B19 in pregnancy can lead to several complications, particularly in the first and second trimesters. Complications are:
- Miscarriage or fetal death
- Severe fetal anaemia
- **Hydrops fetalis** (fetal heart failure)
- Maternal pre-eclampsia-like syndrome

Fetal anaemia is caused by parvovirus infection of the **erythroid progenitor cells** in the fetal **bone marrow** and **liver**. These cells produce **red blood cells**, and the infection causes them to produce faulty red blood cells that have a shorter life span. Less red blood cells results in anaemia. This anaemia leads to heart failure, referred to as **hydrops fetalis**.

Maternal pre-eclampsia-like syndrome is also known as **mirror syndrome**. It can be a rare complication of severe fetal heart failure (**hydrops fetalis**). It involves a triad of hydrops fetalis, placental oedema and oedema in the mother. It also features hypertension and proteinuria.

Women suspected of parvovirus infection need tests for:
- IgM to parvovirus, which tests for acute infection within the past four weeks
- IgG to parvovirus, which tests for long term immunity to the virus after a previous infection
- Rubella antibodies (as a differential diagnosis)

Treatment is supportive.

Women with parvovirus B19 infection need a referral to **fetal medicine** to monitor for complications and malformations.

Zika Virus

The zika virus is spread by host **Aedes mosquitos** in areas of the world where the virus is prevalent. It can also be spread by sex with someone infected with the virus. It can cause no symptoms, minimal symptoms, or a mild flu-like illness. In pregnancy, it can lead to **congenital Zika syndrome**, which involves:
- Microcephaly
- Fetal growth restriction
- Other intracranial abnormalities, such as **ventriculomegaly** and **cerebellar atrophy**

Pregnant women that may have contracted the Zika virus should be tested with **viral PCR** and **antibodies to the Zika virus**. Women with a positive result should be referred to **fetal medicine** for close monitoring of the pregnancy. There is no treatment for the virus.

Rhesus Incompatibility

The name **rhesus** refers to various types of **rhesus antigens** on the surface of **red blood cells**. The antigens on the red blood cells vary between individuals. The rhesus antigens are **separate** to the **ABO blood group** system.

Within the rhesus group, many different types of antigens can be present or absent, depending on the person's blood type. The most relevant antigen within the rhesus blood group system is the **rhesus-D antigen**. When we refer to someone's rhesus status in relation to pregnancy (e.g. "she is rhesus-negative"), we are usually referring to whether they have the rhesus-D antigen present on their red blood cell surface.

Rhesus Incompatibility in Pregnancy

Women that are **rhesus-D positive** do not need any additional treatment during pregnancy.

When a woman that is **rhesus-D negative** becomes pregnant, we have to consider the possibility that her child will be **rhesus positive**. It is likely at some point in the pregnancy (i.e. childbirth) that the blood from the baby will find a way into the mother's bloodstream. When this happens, the baby's **red blood cells** display the **rhesus-D antigen**. The mother's immune system will recognise this rhesus-D antigen as foreign, and produce **antibodies** to the rhesus-D antigen. The mother has then become **sensitised** to rhesus-D antigens.

Usually, this sensitisation process does not cause problems during the first pregnancy. During subsequent pregnancies, the mother's anti-rhesus-D antibodies can cross the placenta into the fetus. If that fetus is rhesus-D positive, these antibodies attach themselves to the red blood cells of the fetus and causes the immune system of the fetus to attack them, causing destruction of the red blood cells (**haemolysis**). The red blood cell destruction caused by antibodies from the mother is called **haemolytic disease of the newborn**.

Management

Prevention of sensitisation is the mainstay of management. This involves giving intramuscular **anti-D** injections to rhesus-D negative women. There is no way to reverse the sensitisation process once it has occurred, which is why prophylaxis is so essential.

The **anti-D** medication works by attaching itself to the rhesus-D antigens on the fetal red blood cells in the mother's circulation, causing them to be destroyed. This prevents the mother's immune system recognising the antigen and creating it's own antibodies to the antigen. It acts to prevent the mother becoming sensitised to the rhesus-D antigen.

Anti-D injections are given routinely on two occasions:
- 28 weeks gestation
- Birth (if the baby's blood group is found to be rhesus-positive)

Anti-D injections should also be given at any time where sensitisation may occur, such as:
- Antepartum haemorrhage
- Amniocentesis procedures
- Abdominal trauma

Anti-D is given within 72 hours of a sensitisation event. After 20 weeks gestation, the **Kleinhauer test** is performed to see how much fetal blood has passed into the mother's blood, to determine whether further doses of anti-D are required.

Kleihauer Test

The Kleihauer test checks how much fetal blood has passed into the mother's blood during a sensitisation event. This test is used after any sensitising event past 20 weeks gestation, to assess whether further doses of anti-D are required.

The Kleihauer test involves adding acid to a sample of the mother's blood. Fetal haemoglobin is naturally more resistant to acid, so that they are protected against the acidosis that occurs around childbirth. Therefore, fetal haemoglobin persists in response to the added acid, while the mothers haemoglobin is destroyed. The number of cells still containing haemoglobin (the remaining fetal cells) can then be calculated.

Small For Gestational Age

Small for gestational age is defined as a fetus that measures below the **10th centile** for their **gestational age**. Two measurements on ultrasound are used to assess the fetal size:
- **Estimated fetal weight (EFW)**
- **Fetal abdominal circumference (AC)**

Customised growth charts are used to assess the size of the fetus, based on the mother's:
- Ethnic group
- Weight
- Height
- Parity

Severe SGA is when the fetus is below the 3rd centile for their gestational age. **Low birth weight** is defined as a birth weight of less than 2500g.

Causes of SGA

The causes of SGA can be divided into two categories:
- **Constitutionally small**, matching the mother and others in the family, and growing appropriately on the growth chart
- **Fetal growth restriction (FGR)**, also known as **intrauterine growth restriction (IUGR)**

Fetal growth restriction (**FGR**), also known as **intrauterine growth restriction** (**IUGR**), is when there is a small fetus (or a fetus that is not growing as expected) due to a pathology reducing the amount of nutrients and oxygen being delivered to the fetus through the placenta.

TOM TIP: It is important to note the difference between small for gestational age (SGA) and fetal growth restriction (FGR). Small for gestational age simply means that the baby is small for the dates, without stating why. The fetus may be constitutionally small, growing appropriately, and not at increased risk of complications. Alternatively, the fetus may be small for gestational age due to pathology (i.e. FGR), with a higher risk of morbidity and mortality.

The causes of **fetal growth restriction** can be divided into two categories:
- **Placenta mediated growth restriction**
- **Non-placenta mediated growth restriction**, where the baby is small due to a genetic or structural abnormality

Placenta mediated growth restriction refers to conditions that affect the transfer of nutrients across the placenta:
- Idiopathic
- Pre-eclampsia
- Maternal smoking
- Maternal alcohol
- Anaemia
- Malnutrition
- Infection
- Maternal health conditions

Non-placenta medicated growth restriction refers to pathology of the fetus, such as:
- Genetic abnormalities
- Structural abnormalities
- Fetal infection
- Errors of metabolism

Other Signs of Fetal Growth Restriction

There may be other signs that would indicate FGR other than the fetus being SGA, such as:
- Reduced amniotic fluid volume
- Abnormal Doppler studies
- Reduced fetal movements
- Abnormal CTGs

Complications

Short term complications of fetal growth restriction include:
- Fetal death or stillbirth
- Birth asphyxia
- Neonatal hypothermia
- Neonatal hypoglycaemia

Growth restricted babies have a long term increased risk of:
- Cardiovascular disease, particularly hypertension
- Type 2 diabetes
- Obesity
- Mood and behavioural problems

Risk Factors

There are a long list of risk factors for SGA:
- Previous SGA baby
- Obesity
- Smoking
- Diabetes
- Existing hypertension
- Pre-eclampsia
- Older mother (over 35 years)
- Multiple pregnancy
- Low pregnancy-associated plasma protein-A (PAPPA)
- Antepartum haemorrhage
- Antiphospholipid syndrome

Monitoring

The **RCOG green-top guidelines** on SGA (2013) lists **major** and **minor** risk factors. At the booking clinic, women are assessed for risk factors for SGA.

Low-risk women have monitoring of the **symphysis fundal height** (**SFH**) at every antenatal appointment from 24 weeks onwards to identify potential SGA. The SFH is plotted on a customised growth chart to assess the appropriate size for the individual woman. If the symphysis fundal height is less than the 10th centile, women are booked for **serial growth scans** with **umbilical artery doppler**.

Women are booked for **serial growth scans** with **umbilical artery Doppler** if they have:
- Three or more minor risk factors
- One or more major risk factors
- Issues with measuring the symphysis fundal height (e.g. large fibroids or BMI > 35)

Women at risk or with SGA are monitored closely with serial ultrasound scans measuring:
- **Estimated fetal weight** (**EFW**) and **abdominal circumference** (**AC**) to determine the **growth velocity**
- **Umbilical arterial pulsatility index** (**UA-PI**) to measure flow through the umbilical artery
- **Amniotic fluid volume**

The local guidelines for the initiation and frequency of ultrasound scans may vary. An example regime is a growth scan every four weeks from 28 weeks gestation. Ultrasound frequency is increased where there is reduced growth velocity or problems with umbilical flow.

Management

The critical management steps are:
- Identifying those at risk of SGA
- Aspirin given to those at risk of pre-eclampsia
- Treating modifiable risk factors (e.g. stop smoking)
- Serial growth scans to monitor growth
- Early delivery where growth is static, or there are other concerns

When a fetus is identified as SGA, investigations to identify the underlying cause include:
- Blood pressure and urine dipstick for pre-eclampsia
- Uterine artery Doppler scanning
- Detailed fetal anatomy scan by **fetal medicine**
- Karyotyping for chromosomal abnormalities
- Testing for infections (e.g. toxoplasmosis, cytomegalovirus, syphilis and malaria)

Early delivery is considered when growth is static on the growth charts, or other problems are identified (e.g. abnormal Doppler results). This reduces the risk of **stillbirth**. **Corticosteroids** are given when delivery is planned early, particularly when delivered by **caesarean section**. Paediatricians should be involved at birth to help with neonatal resuscitation and management if required.

Large for Gestational Age

Babies are defined as being *large for gestational age* (also known as *macrosomia*) when the weight of the newborn is more than **4.5kg at birth**. During pregnancy, an **estimated fetal weight** above the **90th centile** is considered large for gestational age.

Causes of Macrosomia

- Constitutional
- Maternal diabetes
- Previous macrosomia
- Maternal obesity or rapid weight gain
- Overdue
- Male baby

Risks

The risks to the mother include:
- Shoulder dystocia
- Failure to progress
- Perineal tears
- Instrumental delivery or caesarean
- Postpartum haemorrhage
- Uterine rupture (rare)

The risks to the baby include:
- Birth injury (Erbs palsy, clavicular fracture, fetal distress and hypoxia)
- Neonatal hypoglycaemia
- Obesity in childhood and later life
- Type 2 diabetes in adulthood

TOM TIP: If you only remember two things about macrosomia, remember that it is caused by gestational diabetes, and there is a significant risk of shoulder dystocia during birth.

Management

Investigations for a large for gestational age baby are:
- **Ultrasound** to exclude **polyhydramnios** and estimate the **fetal weight**
- **Oral glucose tolerance test** for **gestational diabetes**

Most women with a large for gestational age pregnancy will have a successful vaginal delivery. NICE guidelines (2008) advise against induction of labour only on the grounds of macrosomia.

The main risk with a large for gestational age baby is **shoulder dystocia**. The risks at delivery can be reduced by:
- Delivery on a consultant lead unit
- Delivery by an experienced midwife or obstetrician
- Access to an obstetrician and theatre if required
- Active management of the third stage (delivery of the placenta)
- Early decision for caesarean section if required
- Paediatrician attending the birth

Multiple Pregnancy

Multiple pregnancy refers to a pregnancy with more than one fetus. The incidence of multiple pregnancies increased with the development of fertility treatment.

Types

There are some key definitions to become familiar with relating to twin and multiple pregnancy:
- **Monozygotic**: identical twins (from a single zygote)
- **Dizygotic**: non-identical (from two different zygotes)
- **Monoamniotic**: single amniotic sac
- **Diamniotic**: two separate amniotic sacs
- **Monochorionic**: share a single placenta
- **Dichorionic**: two separate placentas

The best outcomes are with **diamniotic, dichorionic** twin pregnancies, as each fetus has their own nutrient supply.

Diagnosis

Multiple pregnancy is usually diagnosed on the booking ultrasound scan. Ultrasound is also used to determine the:
- Gestational age
- Number of **placentas** (**chorionicity**) and **amniotic sacs** (**amnionicity**)
- Risk of Down's syndrome (as part of the **combined test**)

When determining the type of twins using an ultrasound scan:
- **Dichorionic diamniotic** twins have a membrane between the twins, with a **lambda sign** or **twin peak sign**
- **Monochorionic diamniotic** twins have a membrane between the twins, with a **T sign**
- **Monochorionic monoamniotic** twins have no membrane separating the twins

The **lambda sign**, or **twin peak sign**, refers to a triangular appearance where the **membrane** between the twins meets the **chorion**, as the chorion blends partially into the membrane. This indicates a dichorionic twin pregnancy (separate placentas).

The **T sign** refers to where the membrane between the twins abruptly meets the chorion, giving a T appearance. This indicates a monochorionic twin pregnancy (single placenta).

Complications

Risks to the mother:
- Anaemia
- Polyhydramnios
- Hypertension
- Malpresentation
- Spontaneous preterm birth
- Instrumental delivery or caesarean
- Postpartum haemorrhage

Risks to the fetuses and neonates:
- Miscarriage
- Stillbirth
- Fetal growth restriction
- Prematurity
- Twin-twin transfusion syndrome
- Twin anaemia polycythaemia sequence
- Congenital abnormalities

Twin-Twin Transfusion Syndrome

Twin-twin transfusion syndrome occurs when the fetuses share a placenta. It is called **feto-fetal transfusion syndrome** in pregnancies with more than two fetuses.

When there is a connection between the blood supplies of the two fetuses, one fetus (the **recipient**) may receive the majority of the blood from the placenta, while the other fetus (the **donor**) is starved of blood. The **recipient** gets the majority of the blood, and can become fluid overloaded, with **heart failure** and **polyhydramnios**. The donor has **growth restriction**, **anaemia** and **oligohydramnios**. There will be a discrepancy between the size of the fetuses.

Women with twin-twin transfusion syndrome need to be referred to a tertiary specialist fetal medicine centre. In severe cases, **laser treatment** may be used to destroy the connection between the two blood supplies.

Twin Anaemia Polycythaemia Sequence

Twin anaemia polycythaemia sequence is similar to twin-twin transfusion syndrome, but less acute. One twin becomes **anaemic** whilst the other develops **polycythaemia** (raised haemoglobin).

Antenatal Care

The NICE guidelines (2019) on multiple pregnancy advise about additional management for multiple pregnancies. A specialist multiple pregnancy obstetric team manages women with multiple pregnancy.

Women with multiple pregnancy require additional monitoring for **anaemia**, with a **full blood count** at:
- Booking clinic
- 20 weeks gestation
- 28 weeks gestation

Additional ultrasound scans are required in multiple pregnancy to monitor for **fetal growth restriction**, **unequal growth** and **twin-twin transfusion syndrome**:
- 2 weekly scans from 16 weeks for monochorionic twins
- 4 weekly scans from 20 weeks for dichorionic twins

Planned birth is offered between:
- 32 and 33 + 6 weeks for uncomplicated monochorionic monoamniotic twins
- 36 and 36 + 6 weeks for uncomplicated monochorionic diamniotic twins
- 37 and 37 + 6 weeks for uncomplicated dichorionic diamniotic twins
- Before 35 + 6 weeks for triplets

Waiting beyond these dates is associated with an increased risk of fetal death. The timing of birth when there are complications is assessed on an individual basis. **Corticosteroids** are given before delivery to help mature the lungs.

Delivery

Monoamniotic twins require **elective caesarean section** at between 32 and 33 + 6 weeks.

Diamniotic twins (aim to deliver between 37 and 37 + 6 weeks):
- **Vaginal delivery** is possible when the first baby has a **cephalic presentation** (head first)
- **Caesarean section** may be required for the second baby after successful birth of the first baby
- **Elective caesarean** is advised when the presenting twin is **not** cephalic presentation

Urinary Tract Infection in Pregnancy

Lower urinary tract infection involves infection in the bladder, causing **cystitis** (inflammation of the bladder). **Upper urinary tract infection** involves infection up to the kidneys, called **pyelonephritis**.

Pregnant women are at higher risk of developing lower urinary tract infections and pyelonephritis.

Urinary tract infections in pregnant women increase the risk of **preterm delivery**. They may also increase the risk of other adverse pregnancy outcomes, such as low birth weight and pre-eclampsia.

Asymptomatic Bacteriuria

Asymptomatic bacteriuria refers to bacteria present in the urine, without symptoms of infection. Pregnant women with asymptomatic bacteriuria are at higher risk of developing **lower urinary tract infections** and **pyelonephritis**, and subsequently at risk of **preterm birth**.

Pregnant women are tested for **asymptomatic bacteriuria** at booking and routinely throughout pregnancy. This involves sending a urine sample to the lab for **microscopy**, **culture** and **sensitivities** (**MC&S**).

Testing for **bacteria** in the urine of asymptomatic patients is usually not recommended, as it may lead to unnecessary antibiotics. Pregnant women are an exception to this rule, due to the adverse outcomes associated with infection.

Presentation

Lower urinary tract infections present with:
- Dysuria (pain, stinging or burning when passing urine)
- Suprapubic pain or discomfort
- Increased frequency of urination
- Urgency
- Incontinence
- Haematuria

Pyelonephritis presents with:
- **Fever** (more prominent than in lower urinary tract infections)
- **Loin**, **suprapubic** or **back pain** (this may be bilateral or unilateral)
- Looking and feeling generally unwell
- Vomiting
- Loss of appetite
- Haematuria
- Renal angle tenderness on examination

Urine Dipstick

Nitrites are produced by gram-negative bacteria (such as **E. coli**). These bacteria break down **nitrates**, a normal waste product in urine, into **nitrites**. The nitrites in the urine suggest the presence of bacteria.

Leukocytes refer to **white blood cells**. There are normally a small number of leukocytes in the urine, but a significant rise can be the result of an infection, or alternative cause of inflammation. Urine dipstick tests examine for **leukocyte esterase**, a product of leukocytes, which gives an indication of the number of leukocytes in the urine.

Nitrites are a more accurate indication of infection than **leukocytes**.

During pregnancy, **midstream urine** (**MSU**) samples are routinely sent to the microbiology lab to be cultured and to have sensitivity testing.

Causes

Most common cause of urinary tract infection is **Escherichia coli** (**E. coli**). This is a gram-negative, anaerobic, rod-shaped bacteria that is part of the normal lower intestinal microbiome. It is found in faeces, and can easily spread to the bladder.

Other causes:
- **Klebsiella pneumoniae** (gram-negative anaerobic rod)
- Enterococcus
- Pseudomonas aeruginosa
- Staphylococcus saprophyticus
- Candida albicans (fungal)

Management

Urinary tract infection in pregnancy requires **7 days** of antibiotics.

The antibiotic options are:
- Nitrofurantoin (avoid in the third trimester)
- Amoxicillin (only after sensitivities are known)
- Cefalexin

Nitrofurantoin needs to be avoided in the **third trimester** as there is a risk of **neonatal haemolysis** (destruction of the neonatal red blood cells).

Trimethoprim needs to be avoided in the **first trimester** as it is works as a **folate antagonist**. Folate is important in early pregnancy for the normal development of the fetus. Trimethoprim in early pregnancy can cause **congenital malformations**, particularly **neural tube defects** (i.e. **spina bifida**). It is not known to be harmful later in pregnancy, but is generally avoided unless necessary.

Anaemia in Pregnancy

Anaemia is defined as a low concentration of **haemoglobin** in the blood. This is the result of an underlying disease and is not a disease itself. The prefix **an-** means without, and the suffix **–aemia** relates to blood.

Haemoglobin is a protein found in **red blood cells**. It is responsible for picking up **oxygen** in the lungs and transporting it to the cells of the body. **Iron** is an essential ingredient in creating **haemoglobin** and forms part of the structure of the molecule.

Women are routinely screened for anaemia twice during pregnancy:
- Booking clinic
- 28 weeks gestation

During pregnancy, the **plasma volume** increases. This results in a reduction in the **haemoglobin concentration**. The blood is diluted due to the higher plasma volume.

It is important to optimise the treatment of anaemia during pregnancy so that the woman has reasonable reserves, in case there is significant blood loss during delivery.

Presentation

Often anaemia in pregnancy is asymptomatic. Women may have:
- Shortness of breath
- Fatigue
- Dizziness
- Pallor

Investigations

The normal ranges for haemoglobin during pregnancy are:

Time	Haemoglobin Concentration
Booking bloods	> 110 g/l
28 weeks gestation	> 105 g/l
Post partum	> 100 g/l

The **mean cell volume** (**MCV**) can indicate the cause of the anaemia:
- Low MCV may indicate **iron deficiency**
- Normal MCV may indicate a **physiological anaemia** due to the increased plasma volume of pregnancy
- Raised MCV may indicate **B12** or **folate deficiency**

Women are offered **haemoglobinopathy screening** at the booking clinic for **thalassaemia** (all women) and **sickle cell disease** (women at higher risk). Both are causes of significant anaemia in pregnancy.

Additional investigations are **not** routinely performed, by may help establish the cause of the anaemia. They may include:
- Ferritin
- B12
- Folate

Management

Iron
Women with anaemia in pregnancy are started on iron replacement (e.g. ferrous sulphate 200mg three times daily). When women are not anaemic, but have a low ferritin (indicating low iron stores), they may be started on supplementary iron.

B12

The increased plasma volume and B12 requirements often result in a low B12 in pregnancy. Women with low B12 should be tested for **pernicious anaemia** (checking for **intrinsic factor antibodies**).

Advice should be sought from a haematologist regarding further investigations and treatment of low B12 in pregnancy. Treatment options for low B12 are:
- Intramuscular **hydroxocobalamin** injections
- Oral **cyanocobalamin** tablets

Folate

All women should already be taking folic acid 400mcg per day. Women with folate deficiency are started on folic acid 5mg daily.

Thalassaemia and Sickle Cell Anaemia

Women with a haemoglobinopathy will be managed jointly with a specialist haematologist. They require high dose folic acid (5mg), close monitoring and transfusions when required.

Venous Thromboembolism in Pregnancy

Venous thromboembolism (**VTE**) is a common and potentially fatal condition. It involves blood clots (**thrombosis**) developing in the circulation. Thrombosis occurs as a result of **stagnation of blood**, and **hyper-coagulable** states, such as pregnancy.

When a **thrombosis** develops in the venous circulation, it is called **deep vein thrombosis** (**DVT**). This thrombosis can mobilise (**embolisation**) from the deep veins and travel to the lungs, where it becomes lodged in the **pulmonary arteries**. This blocks blood flow to related areas of the lungs, and is called a **pulmonary embolism** (**PE**).

Pulmonary embolism is a significant cause of death in obstetrics. The risk is significantly reduced with **VTE prophylaxis**. The risk is highest in the postpartum period.

Risk Factors

There is a long list of risk factors for VTE in pregnancy:
- Smoking
- Parity ≥ 3
- Age > 35 years
- BMI > 30
- Reduced mobility
- Multiple pregnancy
- Pre-eclampsia
- Gross varicose veins
- Immobility
- Family history of VTE
- Thrombophilia
- IVF pregnancy

The RCOG guidelines (2015) advise starting prophylaxis from:
- **First trimester** if there are **three** risk factors
- **28 weeks** if there are **four or more** of these risk factors

There are additional scenarios where prophylaxis is considered, even in the absence of other risk factors:
- Hospital admission
- Surgical procedures
- Previous VTE
- Medical conditions such as cancer or arthritis
- High-risk thrombophilias
- Ovarian hyperstimulation syndrome

VTE Prophylaxis

All pregnant women should have a risk assessment for their risk of **venous thromboembolism** (**VTE**) at booking. A risk assessment is performed again after birth. Additional risk assessments are necessary at other times, such as if they are admitted to hospital, undergo a procedure or develop significant immobility. Each unit will have a policy and protocol for assessing risk and starting prophylaxis in pregnancy.

Women at increased risk of VTE should receive prophylaxis with **low molecular weight heparin** (**LMWH**) unless contraindicated. Examples of LMWH are **enoxaparin**, **dalteparin** and **tinzaparin**. Prophylaxis is started as soon as possible in very high risk patients and at 28 weeks in those at high risk. It is continued throughout the antenatal period and for six weeks postnatally.

Prophylaxis is temporarily stopped when the woman goes into labour, and can be started immediately after delivery (except with postpartum haemorrhage, spinal anaesthesia and epidurals).

Mechanical prophylaxis may be considered in women with contraindications to LMWH. The options for mechanical prophylaxis are:
- *Intermittent pneumatic compression* with equipment that inflates and deflates to massage the legs
- *Anti-embolic compression stockings*

Presentation

Deep vein thrombosis is almost always **unilateral**. Bilateral DVTs are rare, and bilateral symptoms are more likely due to an alternative diagnosis, such as **chronic venous** or **pre-eclampsia**. DVTs present with:
- Calf or leg swelling
- Dilated superficial veins
- Tenderness to the calf (particularly over the deep veins)
- Oedema
- Colour changes to the leg

To examine for leg swelling measure the circumference of the calf 10cm below the **tibial tuberosity**. **More than 3cm** difference between calves is significant.

Pulmonary embolism can present with subtle signs and symptoms. In patients with potential features of a PE, risk factors for PE, and no other explanation for their symptoms, have a low threshold for suspecting a PE. Presenting features include:
- Shortness of breath
- Cough with or without blood (**haemoptysis**)
- Pleuritic chest pain
- Hypoxia
- Tachycardia (this can be difficult to distinguish from the normal physiological changes in pregnancy)
- Raised respiratory rate
- Low-grade fever
- Haemodynamic instability causing hypotension

Diagnosis

Doppler ultrasound is the investigation of choice for patients with suspected **deep vein thrombosis**. The RCOG guideline (2015) recommends repeating negative ultrasound scans on day 3 and 7 in patients with a high index of suspicion for DVT.

Women with suspected **pulmonary embolism** require:
- Chest xray
- ECG

There are two main options for establishing a definitive diagnosis of a pulmonary embolism: **CT pulmonary angiogram** (**CTPA**) or **ventilation-perfusion** (**VQ**) scan.

CT pulmonary angiogram involves a chest CT scan with an **intravenous contrast** that highlights the pulmonary arteries to demonstrate any blood clots. This is usually the first choice for investigating a pulmonary embolism, as it tends to be more readily available, provides a more definitive assessment and gives information about alternative diagnoses such as pneumonia or malignancy.

Ventilation-perfusion (VQ) scan involves using **radioactive isotopes** and a **gamma camera**, to compare the ventilation with the perfusion of the lungs. First, the isotopes are **inhaled** to fill the lungs, and a picture is taken to demonstrate **ventilation**. Next, a contrast containing isotopes is **injected**, and a picture is taken to demonstrate **perfusion**. The two images are compared. With a pulmonary embolism, there will be a deficit in **perfusion**, as the thrombus blocks blood flow to the lung tissue. This area of lung tissue will be **ventilated** but **not perfused**.

When considering the choice between CTPA and VQ scan:
- CTPA is the test for choice for patients with an abnormal chest xray
- CTPA carries a higher risk of **breast cancer** for the mother (minimal absolute risk)
- VQ scan carries a higher risk of **childhood cancer** for the fetus (minimal absolute risk)

Patients with a suspected **deep vein thrombosis** and **pulmonary embolism** should have a **Doppler ultrasound** initially, and if a DVT is present, they do **not** require a VQ scan or CTPA to confirm a PE. The treatment for DVT and PE are the same.

TOM TIP: The Wells score is not validated for use in pregnant women. D-dimers are not helpful in pregnant patients, as pregnancy is a cause of a raised D-dimer.

Management

Management of **venous thromboembolism** in pregnancy is with **low molecular weight heparin** (**LMWH**). Examples of LMWH are **enoxaparin**, **dalteparin** and **tinzaparin**. The dose is based on the woman's **weight** at the **booking clinic**, or from early pregnancy.

LMWH should be started immediately, **before** confirming the diagnosis in patients where DVT or PE is suspected and there is a delay in getting the scan. Treatment can be stopped when the investigations **exclude** the diagnosis.

When the diagnosis is confirmed, LMWH is continued for the remained of pregnancy plus six weeks postnatally, or three months in total (whichever is longer). There is an option to switch to **oral anticoagulation** (e.g. warfarin or a DOAC) after delivery. An individual risk assessment is performed before stopping anticoagulation, with advice from a haematologist if necessary.

Women with a ***massive PE*** and ***haemodynamic compromise*** need immediate management by an experienced team of medical doctors, obstetricians, radiologists and others. This is a life-threatening scenario. Treatment options are:
- Unfractionated heparin
- Thrombolysis
- Surgical embolectomy

Pre-eclampsia

Pre-eclampsia refers to new high blood pressure (***hypertension***) in pregnancy with **end-organ dysfunction**, notably with ***proteinuria*** (protein in the urine). It occurs **after 20 weeks** gestation, when the **spiral arteries** of the placenta form abnormally, leading to a **high vascular resistance** in these vessels.

Pre-eclampsia is a significant cause of maternal and fetal morbidity and mortality. Without treatment, it can lead to maternal organ damage, fetal growth restriction, seizures, early labour and in a small proportion, death.

Pre-eclampsia features a triad of:
- Hypertension
- Proteinuria
- Oedema

Definitions

Chronic hypertension is high blood pressure that exists before 20 weeks gestation and is longstanding. This is not caused by dysfunction in the placenta and is not classed as pre-eclampsia.

Pregnancy-induced hypertension or ***gestational hypertension*** is hypertension occurring after 20 weeks gestation, without proteinuria.

Pre-eclampsia is pregnancy-induced hypertension associated with organ damage, notably ***proteinuria***.

Eclampsia is when ***seizures*** occur as a result of pre-eclampsia.

Pathophysiology

The pathophysiology of pre-eclampsia is poorly understood. The following is a simplified explanation.

When the ***blastocyst*** implants on the ***endometrium***, the outermost layer, called the ***syncytiotrophoblast***, grows into the endometrium. It forms finger-like projections called chorionic villi. The chorionic villi contain fetal blood vessels.

Trophoblast invasion of the endometrium sends signals to the ***spiral arteries*** in that area of the endometrium, reducing their ***vascular resistance*** and making them more fragile. The blood flow to these arteries increases, and eventually they break down, leaving pools of blood called ***lacunae*** (lakes). Maternal blood flows from the uterine arteries, into these lacunae, and back out through the uterine veins. Lacunae form at around 20 weeks gestation.

When the process of forming lacunae is inadequate, the woman can develop pre-eclampsia. Pre-eclampsia is caused by **high vascular resistance** in the **spiral arteries** and **poor perfusion** of the placenta. This causes **oxidative stress** in the placenta, and the release of inflammatory chemicals into the systemic circulation, leading to **systemic inflammation** and **impaired endothelial function** in the blood vessels.

Risk Factors

The NICE guidelines categorise the risk factors into **high-risk** and **moderate-risk factors**.

High-risk factors are:
- Pre-existing hypertension
- Previous hypertension in pregnancy
- Existing autoimmune conditions (e.g. systemic lupus erythematosus)
- Diabetes
- Chronic kidney disease

Moderate-risk factors are:
- Older than 40
- BMI > 35
- More than 10 years since previous pregnancy
- Multiple pregnancy
- First pregnancy
- Family history of pre-eclampsia

These risk factors are used to determine which women are offered aspirin as prophylaxis against pre-eclampsia. Women are offered aspirin from 12 weeks gestation until birth if they have **one high-risk factor** or **more** than one **moderate-risk factors**.

Symptoms

Pre-eclampsia has symptoms of the complications:
- Headache
- Visual disturbance or blurriness
- Nausea and vomiting
- Upper abdominal or epigastric pain (this is due to liver swelling)
- Oedema
- Reduced urine output
- Brisk reflexes

Diagnosis

The NICE guidelines (2019) advise a diagnosis can be made with a:
- Systolic blood pressure above 140 mmHg
- Diastolic blood pressure above 90 mmHg

PLUS any of:
- **Proteinuria** (1+ or more on urine dipstick)
- **Organ dysfunction** (e.g. raised creatinine, elevated liver enzymes, seizures, thrombocytopenia or haemolytic anaemia)
- **Placental dysfunction** (e.g. fetal growth restriction or abnormal Doppler studies)

Proteinuria can be quantified using:
- *Urine albumin:creatinine ratio* (above 30mg/mmol is significant)
- *Urine protein:creatinine ratio* (above 8mg/mmol is significant)

The NICE guidelines (2019) recommend the use of **placental growth factor** (**PlGF**) testing on one occasion during pregnancy in women suspected of having pre-eclampsia. **Placental growth factor** is a **protein** released by the placenta that functions to stimulate the development of new blood vessels. In pre-eclampsia, the levels of PlGF are low. NICE recommends using PlGF between 20 and 35 weeks gestation to **rule-out** pre-eclampsia.

Management

Aspirin is used for prophylaxis against the development of pre-eclampsia. It is given from 12 weeks gestation until birth to women with:
- A single **high-risk** factor
- Two or more **moderate-risk** factors

All pregnant women are routinely monitored at every antenatal appointment for evidence of pre-eclampsia, with:
- Blood pressure
- Symptoms
- Urine dipstick for proteinuria

When gestational hypertension (without proteinuria) is identified, the general management involves:
- Treating to aim for a blood pressure below 135/85 mmHg
- Admission for women with a blood pressure above 160/110 mmHg
- Urine dipstick testing at least weekly
- Monitoring of blood tests weekly (full blood count, liver enzymes and renal profile)
- Monitoring fetal growth by serial growth scans
- PlGF testing on one occasion

When pre-eclampsia is diagnosed, the general management is similar to gestational diabetes, except:
- Scoring systems are used to determine whether to admit the woman (**fullPIERS** or **PREP-S**)
- Blood pressure is monitored closely (at least every 48 hours)
- Urine dipstick testing is not routinely necessary (the diagnosis is already made)
- Ultrasound monitoring of the fetus, amniotic fluid and Dopplers is performed two weekly

Medical management of pre-eclampsia is with:
- **Labetolol** is first-line as an antihypertensive
- **Nifedipine** (modified-release) is commonly used second-line
- **Methyldopa** is used third-line (needs to be stopped within two days of birth)
- **Intravenous hydralazine** may be used as an antihypertensive in critical care in **severe pre-eclampsia** or **eclampsia**
- **IV magnesium sulphate** is given during labour and in the 24 hours afterwards to prevent seizures
- **Fluid restriction** is used during labour in **severe pre-eclampsia** or **eclampsia**, to avoid fluid overload

Planned early birth may be necessary if the blood pressure cannot be controlled or complications occur. **Corticosteroids** should be given to women having a premature birth to help mature the fetal lungs.

Blood pressure is monitored closely after delivery. Blood pressure will return to normal over time once the placenta is removed.

For medical treatment **after delivery**, NICE recommend switching to one or a combination of:
1. Enalapril (first-line)
2. Nifedipine or amlodipine (first-line in black African or Caribbean patients)
3. Labetolol or atenolol (third-line)

Eclampsia

Eclampsia refers to the seizures associated with pre-eclampsia. **IV magnesium sulphate** is used to manage seizures associated with pre-eclampsia.

HELLP Syndrome

HELLP syndrome is a combination of features that occurs as a complication of pre-eclampsia and eclampsia. It is an acronym for the key characteristics:
- **H**aemolysis
- **E**levated **L**iver enzymes
- **L**ow **P**latelets

Gestational Diabetes

Gestational diabetes refers to diabetes triggered by pregnancy. It is caused by **reduced insulin sensitivity** during pregnancy, and resolves after birth.

The most significant immediate complication of gestational diabetes is a **large for dates** fetus and **macrosomia**. This has implications for birth, mainly posing a risk of **shoulder dystocia**. Longer term, women are at higher risk of developing **type 2 diabetes**.

Anyone with **risk factors** should be screened with an **oral glucose tolerance test** at 24 - 28 weeks gestation. Women with previous gestational diabetes also have an OGTT soon after the booking clinic.

Risk Factors

The NICE guidelines (2015) list the risk factors that warrant testing for gestational diabetes:
- Previous gestational diabetes
- Previous macrosomic baby (≥ 4.5kg)
- BMI > 30
- Ethnic origin (black Caribbean, Middle Eastern and South Asian)
- Family history of diabetes (first-degree relative)

Oral Glucose Tolerance Test

The screening test of choice for gestational diabetes is an **oral glucose tolerance test** (**OGTT**). An OGTT is used in patients with **risk factors** for gestational diabetes, and also when there are features that suggest gestational diabetes:
- Large for dates fetus
- Polyhydramnios (increased amniotic fluid)
- Glucose on urine dipstick

An OGTT should be performed in the morning after a fast (they can drink plain water). The patient has a **75g glucose** drink at the start of the test. The blood sugar level is measured before the sugar drink (**fasting**) and then at **2 hours**.

Normal results are:
- Fasting: < 5.6 mmol/l
- At 2 hours: < 7.8 mmol/l

Results higher than these values are used to diagnose **gestational diabetes**.

TOM TIP: It is really easy to remember the cutoff for gestational diabetes as simply 5 - 6 - 7 - 8.

Management

Patients with gestational diabetes are managed in joint diabetes and antenatal clinics, with input from a dietician. Women need careful explanation about the condition, and to learn how to monitor and track their blood sugar levels. They need four weekly ultrasound scans to monitor the fetal growth and amniotic fluid volume from 28 to 36 weeks gestation.

The initial management suggested by the NICE guidelines (2015) is:
- Fasting glucose less than 7 mmol/l: trial of **diet and exercise** for 1-2 weeks, followed by **metformin**, then **insulin**
- Fasting glucose above 7 mmol/l: start **insulin ± metformin**
- Fasting glucose above 6 mmol/l plus **macrosomia** (or other complications): start **insulin ± metformin**

Glibenclamide (a **sulfonylurea**) is suggested as an option for women who decline insulin or cannot tolerate metformin.

Women need to monitor their blood sugar levels several times a day. The NICE (2015) target levels are:
- Fasting: 5.3 mmol/l
- 1 hour post-meal: 7.8 mmol/l
- 2 hours post-meal: 6.4 mmol/l
- Avoiding levels of 4 mmol/l or below

Pre-Existing Diabetes

Before becoming pregnant, women with existing diabetes should aim for good glucose control. They should take **5mg folic acid** from preconception until 12 weeks gestation.

Women with existing **type 1** and **type 2 diabetes** should aim for the same target insulin levels as with gestational diabetes. Women with type 2 diabetes are managed using **metformin** and **insulin**, and other oral diabetic medications should be stopped.

Retinopathy screening should be performed shortly after booking and at 28 weeks gestation. This involves referral to an **ophthalmologist** to check for **diabetic retinopathy**. Diabetes carries a risk of rapid progression of retinopathy, and interventions may be required.

NICE (2015) advise a **planned delivery** between 37 and 38 + 6 weeks for women with pre-existing diabetes. (Women with gestational diabetes can give birth up to 40 + 6).

A **sliding-scale insulin regime** is considered during labour for women with type 1 diabetes. A **dextrose** and **insulin infusion** is titrated to blood sugar levels, according to the local protocol. This is also considered for women with **poorly controlled** blood sugars with gestational or type 2 diabetes.

TOM TIP: It is worth remembering the importance of retinopathy screening during pregnancy for women with existing diabetes. This is an exam favourite, and will score you extra points with your seniors if you mention it in the antenatal clinic.

Postnatal Care

Diabetes improves immediately after birth. Women with gestational diabetes can stop their diabetic medications immediately after birth. They need follow up to test their fasting glucose after at least six weeks.

Women with existing diabetes should lower their insulin doses and be wary of **hypoglycaemia** in the postnatal period. The insulin sensitivity will increase after birth and with breastfeeding.

Babies of mothers with diabetes are at risk of:
- Neonatal hypoglycaemia
- Polycythaemia (raised haemoglobin)
- Jaundice (raised bilirubin)
- Congenital heart disease
- Cardiomyopathy

Babies need close monitoring for **neonatal hypoglycaemia**, with regular blood glucose checks and frequent feeds. The aim is to maintain their blood sugar above 2 mmol/l, and if it falls below this, they may need **IV dextrose** or **nasogastric feeding**.

TOM TIP: If you remember two complications of gestational diabetes, remember macrosomia and neonatal hypoglycaemia. Babies become accustomed to a large supply of glucose during the pregnancy, and after birth they struggle to maintain the supply they are used to with oral feeding alone.

Obstetric Cholestasis

Obstetric cholestasis is also known as **intrahepatic cholestasis of pregnancy**. **Chole-** relates to the bile and bile ducts. **Stasis** refers to inactivity. Obstetric cholestasis is characterised by the reduced outflow of **bile acids** from the liver. The condition resolves after delivery of the baby.

Obstetric cholestasis is a relatively common complication of pregnancy, occurring in around 1% of pregnant women. It usually develops later in pregnancy (i.e. after 28 weeks), and is thought to be the result of increased **oestrogen** and **progesterone** levels. There seems to be a genetic component. It is more common in women of South Asian ethnicity.

Bile acids are produced in the liver from the breakdown of **cholesterol**. Bile acids flow from liver to the **hepatic ducts**, past the **gallbladder** and out of the **bile duct** to the intestines. In obstetric cholestasis, the outflow of bile acids is reduced, causing them to build up in the blood, resulting in the classic symptoms of itching (**pruritis**).

Obstetric cholestasis is associated with an increased risk of **stillbirth**.

Presentation

Obstetric cholestasis typically present later in pregnancy, particularly in the third trimester.

Itching (*pruritis*) is the main symptom, particularly affecting the **palms of the hands** and **soles of the feet**.

Other symptoms are related to cholestasis and outflow obstruction in the bile ducts:
- Fatigue
- Dark urine
- Pale, greasy stools
- Jaundice

Importantly, there is no rash associated with obstetric cholestasis. If a rash is present, an alternative diagnosis should be considered, such as **polymorphic eruption of pregnancy** or **pemphigoid gestationis**.

Differential Diagnosis

Other causes of pruritus and deranged LFTs should be excluded, for example:
- Gallstones
- Acute fatty liver
- Autoimmune hepatitis
- Viral hepatitis

Investigations

Women presenting with pruritus should have **liver function tests** and **bile acids** checked.

Obstetric cholestasis will cause:
- Abnormal liver function tests (LFTs), mainly ALT, AST and GGT
- Raised bile acids

TOM TIP: It is normal for alkaline phosphatase (ALP) to increase in pregnancy. This is because the placenta produces ALP. A rise in ALP without other abnormal LFT results is usually due to placental production of ALP, rather than liver pathology.

Management

Ursodeoxycholic acid is the primary treatment for obstetric cholestasis. It improves LFTs, bile acids and symptoms.

Symptoms of itching can be managed with:
- **Emollients** (i.e. **calamine lotion**) to soothe the skin
- **Antihistamines** (e.g. **chlorphenamine**) can help **sleeping** (but does not improve itching)

Water-soluble vitamin K can be given if clotting (**prothrombin time**) is deranged. Vitamin K is a fat-soluble vitamin. Bile acids are important in the absorption of fat-soluble vitamins in the intestines. A lack of bile acids can lead to vitamin K deficiency. Vitamin K is an important part of the clotting system, and deficiency can lead to impaired clotting of blood.

Monitoring of LFTs is required during pregnancy (weekly) and after delivery (after at least ten days), to ensure the condition does not worsen and resolves after birth.

Planned delivery after 37 weeks may be considered, particularly when the LFTs and bile acids are severely deranged. Stillbirth in obstetric cholestasis is difficult to predict, and early delivery aims to reduce the risk.

Acute Fatty Liver of Pregnancy

Acute fatty liver of pregnancy is a rare condition that occurs in the **third trimester** of pregnancy. There is a rapid accumulation of fat within the liver cells (**hepatocytes**), causing **acute hepatitis**. There is a high risk of **liver failure** and **mortality**, for both the mother and fetus.

Pathophysiology

Acute fatty liver of pregnancy results from impaired processing of **fatty acids** in the **placenta**. This is the result of a genetic condition in the fetus that impairs fatty acid metabolism. The most common cause is **long-chain 3-hydroxyacyl-CoA dehydrogenase (LCHAD) deficiency** in the fetus, which is an **autosomal recessive** condition. This mode of inheritance means the mother will also have one defective copy of the gene.

Th **LCHAD enzyme** is important in **fatty acid oxidation**, breaking down fatty acids to be used as fuel. The fetus and placenta are unable to break down fatty acids. These fatty acids enter the maternal circulation, and accumulate in the liver. The mother's defective copy of the gene may also contribute to the accumulation of fatty acids. The accumulation of fatty acids in the mother's liver leads to inflammation and liver failure.

Presentation

The presentation is with vague symptoms associated with hepatitis :
- General malaise and fatigue
- Nausea and vomiting
- Jaundice
- Abdominal pain
- Anorexia (lack of appetite)
- **Ascites**

Bloods

Liver function tests will show elevated liver enzymes (**ALT** and **AST**).

Other bloods may be deranged, with:
- Raised bilirubin
- Raised WBC count
- Deranged clotting (raised prothrombin time and INR)
- Low platelets

TOM TIP: In your exams, elevated liver enzymes and low platelets should make you think of HELLP syndrome rather than acute fatty liver of pregnancy. HELLP syndrome is much more common, but keep acute fatty liver of pregnancy in mind as a differential.

Management

Acute fatty liver of pregnancy is an **obstetric emergency** and requires prompt admission and **delivery** of the baby. Most patients will recover after delivery.

Management also involves treatment of **acute liver failure** if it occurs, including consideration of **liver transplant.**

Pregnancy-Related Rashes

There are several pregnancy-related skin changes and rashes that can occur. This section goes through some of the key ones to remember for your exams.

Polymorphic Eruption of Pregnancy

Polymorphic eruption of pregnancy is also known as **pruritic and urticarial papules and plaques of pregnancy**. It is an itchy rash that tends to start in the **third trimester**. It usually begins on the **abdomen**, particularly associated with stretch marks (**striae**).

It is characterised by:
- **Urticarial papules** (raised itchy lumps)
- **Wheals** (raised itchy areas of skin)
- **Plaques** (larger inflamed areas of skin)

The condition will get better towards the end of pregnancy and after delivery. Management is to control the symptoms, with:
- Topical emollients
- Topical steroids
- Oral antihistamines
- Oral steroids may be used in severe cases

Atopic Eruption of Pregnancy

Atopic eruption of pregnancy essentially refers to eczema that flares up during pregnancy. This includes both women that have never suffered with eczema and those with pre-existing eczema. Atopic eruption of pregnancy presents in the **first and second trimester** of pregnancy.

There are two types:
- **E-type**, or **eczema-type**: with eczematous, inflamed, red and itchy skin, typically affecting the insides of the elbows, back of knees, neck, face and chest.
- **P-type**, or **prurigo-type**: with intensely itchy papules (spots) typically affecting the abdomen, back and limbs.

The condition will usually get better after delivery.

Management is with:
- Topical emollients
- Topical steroids
- Phototherapy with ultraviolet light (UVB) may be used in severe cases
- Oral steroids may be used in severe cases

Melasma

Melasma is also known as **mask of pregnancy**. It is characterised by **increased pigmentation** to patches of the skin on the face. This is usually symmetrical and flat, affecting sun-exposed areas.

Melasma is thought to be partly related to the increased female sex hormones associated with pregnancy. It can also occur with the **combined contraceptive pill** and **hormone replacement therapy**. It is also associated with sun exposure, thyroid disease and family history.

No active treatment is required if the appearance is acceptable to the woman. Management is with:
- Avoiding sun exposure and using suncream
- Makeup (camouflage)
- Skin lightening cream (e.g. hydroquinone or retinoid creams), although not in pregnancy and only under specialist care
- Procedures such as chemical peels or laser treatment (not usually on the NHS)

Pyogenic Granuloma

Pyogenic granuloma is also known as **lobular capillary haemangioma**. This is a benign, rapidly growing tumour of **capillaries**. It present as a discrete lump with a red or dark appearance. They occur more often in pregnancy, and can also be associated with hormonal contraceptives. They can also be triggered by minor trauma or infection.

Pyogenic granuloma present with a rapidly growing lump that develops over days, up to 1-2 cm in size (but can be larger). They often occur on **fingers**, or on the upper chest, back, neck or head. They may cause profuse bleeding and ulceration if injured.

Other differentials, such as malignancy, need to be excluded (particularly **nodular melanoma**). When they occur in pregnancy, they usually resolve without treatment after delivery. Treatment is with **surgical removal** with **histology** to confirm the diagnosis.

Pemphigoid Gestationis

Pemphigoid gestationis is a rare **autoimmune** skin condition that occurs in pregnancy. **Autoantibodies** are created that damage the connection between the **epidermis** and the **dermis**. The pregnant woman's immune system may produce these **antibodies** in response to **placental tissue**. This causes the **epidermis** and **dermis** to separate, creating a space that can fill with fluid, resulting in large fluid-filled blisters (bullae).

Pemphigoid gestationis usually occurs in the second or third trimester. The typical presentation is initially with an itchy red papular or blistering rash around the umbilicus, that then spreads to other parts of the body. Over several weeks, large **fluid-filled blisters** form.

The rash usually resolves without treatment after delivery. It may go through stages of improvement and worsening during pregnancy and after birth. The blisters heal without scarring.

Treatment is with:
- Topical emollients
- Topical steroids
- Oral steroids may be required in severe cases
- Immunosuppressants may be required where steroids are inadequate
- Antibiotics may be necessary if infection occurs

The risks to the baby are:
- Fetal growth restriction
- Preterm delivery
- Blistering rash after delivery (as the maternal antibodies pass to the baby)

Placenta Praevia

Placenta praevia is where the placenta is attached in the lower portion of the uterus, lower than the presenting part of the fetus. **Praevia** directly translates from Latin as "**going before**".

The RCOG guidelines (2018) recommend the following definitions:
- **Low-lying placenta** is used when the placenta is within 20mm of the **internal cervical os**
- **Placenta praevia** is used only when the placenta is **over** the **internal cervical os**

Placenta praevia occurs in around 1% of pregnancies. It is a notable cause of **antepartum haemorrhage**.

TOM TIP: The three causes of antepartum haemorrhage to remember are placenta praevia, placental abruption and vasa praevia. These are serious causes with high morbidity and mortality. Causes of spotting or minor bleeding in pregnancy include cervical ectropion, infection and vaginal abrasions from intercourse or procedures.

Risks

Placenta praevia is associated with increased morbidity and mortality for the mother and fetus. The risks include:
- Antepartum haemorrhage
- Emergency caesarean section
- Emergency hysterectomy
- Maternal anaemia and transfusions
- Preterm birth and low birth weight
- Stillbirth

Grades

Traditionally, there are four grades of placenta praevia. You may still come across these in textbooks and exams:
- **Minor praevia**, or **grade I** - the placenta is in the lower uterus but not reaching the **internal cervical os**
- **Marginal praevia**, or **grade II** - the placenta is reaching, but not covering, the **internal cervical os**
- **Partial praevia**, or **grade III** - the placenta is partially covering the **internal cervical os**
- **Complete praevia**, or **grade IV** - the placenta is completely covering the **internal cervical os**

The RCOG guidelines (2018) recommend **against** using this grading system, as it is considered outdated. The two descriptions used are **low-lying placenta** and **placenta praevia**.

Risk Factors

The risk factors for placenta praevia are:
- Previous caesarean sections
- Previous placenta praevia
- Older maternal age
- Maternal smoking
- Structural uterine abnormalities (e.g. fibroids)
- Assisted reproduction (e.g. IVF)

Presentation and Diagnosis

The 20-week anomaly scan is used to assess the position of the placenta and diagnose placenta praevia.

Many women with placenta praevia are asymptomatic. It may present with painless vaginal bleeding in pregnancy (**antepartum haemorrhage**). Bleeding usually occurs later in pregnancy (around or after 36 weeks).

Management

For women with a low-lying placenta or placenta praevia diagnosed early in pregnancy (e.g. at the 20-week anomaly scan), the RCOG guideline (2018) recommends a repeat transvaginal ultrasound scan at:
- 32 weeks gestation
- 36 weeks gestation (if present on the 32-week scan, to guide decisions about delivery)

Corticosteroids are given between 34 and 35 + 6 weeks gestation to mature the fetal lungs, given the risk of preterm delivery.

Planned delivery is considered between 36 and 37 weeks gestation. It is planned early to reduce the risk of spontaneous **labour** and **bleeding**. **Planned cesarean section** is required with placenta praevia and low-lying placenta (<20mm from the internal os).

Depending on the position of the placenta and fetus, different incisions may be made in the skin and uterus, for example, vertical incisions. **Ultrasound** may be used around the time of the procedure to locate the placenta.

Emergency caesarean section may be required with **premature labour** or **antenatal bleeding**.

The main complication of placenta praevia is **haemorrhage** before, during and after delivery. When this occurs, urgent management is required and may involve:
- Emergency caesarean section
- Blood transfusions
- Intrauterine balloon tamponade
- Uterine artery occlusion
- Emergency hysterectomy

Vasa Praevia

Vasa praevia is a condition where the **fetal vessels** are within the **fetal membranes (chorioamniotic membranes)** and travel across the **internal cervical os**. The **fetal membranes** surround the **amniotic cavity** and developing **fetus**. The fetal vessels consist of the two **umbilical arteries** and single **umbilical vein**.

Vasa translates from Latin as **vessel**. **Praevia** translates from Latin as "**going before**". Vasa praevia is where the vessels are placed over the internal cervical os.

Pathophysiology

Under normal circumstances, the **umbilical cord** containing the fetal vessels (**umbilical arteries** and **vein**) insert directly into the placenta. The fetal vessels are always protected, either by the **umbilical cord** or by the **placenta**. The umbilical cord contains **Wharton's jelly**. Wharton's jelly is a layer of soft connective tissue that surrounds the blood vessels in the umbilical cord, offering protection.

There are two instances where the fetal vessels can be exposed, outside the protection of the umbilical cord or placenta:
- **Velamentous umbilical cord** is where the umbilical cord inserts into the **chorioamniotic membranes**, and the fetal vessels travel unprotected through the membranes before joining the placenta.
- **An accessory lobe** of the **placenta** (also known as a **succenturiate lobe**) will be connected by fetal vessels that travel through the **chorioamniotic membranes** between the placental lobes.

In **vasa praevia**, the **fetal vessels** are exposed, outside the protection of the **umbilical cord** or the **placenta**. The fetal vessels travel through the **chorioamniotic membranes**, and pass across the **internal cervical os** (the inner opening of the cervix). These exposed vessels are prone to bleeding, particularly when the membranes are ruptured during labour and at birth. This can lead to dramatic **fetal blood loss** and **death**.

There are two types of vasa praevia:
- **Type I vasa praevia** - the fetal vessels are exposed as a velamentous umbilical cord
- **Type II vasa praevia** - the fetal vessels are exposed as they travel to an accessory placental lobe

Risk Factors

- Low lying placenta
- IVF pregnancy
- Multiple pregnancy

Presentation

Vasa praevia may be diagnosed by ultrasound during pregnancy. This is the ideal scenario, as it allows a planned caesarean section to reduce the risk of haemorrhage. However, ultrasound is not reliable, and it is often not possible to diagnose antenatally.

It may present with antepartum haemorrhage, with bleeding during the second or third trimester of pregnancy.

It may be detected by vaginal examination during labour, when pulsating fetal vessels in the membranes are seen through the dilated cervix.

Finally, it may be detected during labour when fetal distress and dark-red bleeding occur following rupture of the membranes. This carries a very high **fetal mortality**, even with emergency caesarean section.

Management

For asymptomatic women with vasa praevia, the RCOG guidelines (2018) recommend:
- **Corticosteroids**, given from 32 weeks gestation to mature the fetal lungs
- **Elective caesarean section**, planned for 34 – 36 weeks gestation

Where antepartum haemorrhage occurs, **emergency caesarean section** is required to deliver the fetus before death occurs.

After stillbirth or unexplained fetal compromise during delivery, the placenta is examined for evidence of vasa praevia as a possible cause.

Placental Abruption

Placental abruption refers to when the placenta separates from the wall of the uterus during pregnancy. The site of attachment can bleed extensively after the placenta separates. Placental abruption is a significant cause of **antepartum haemorrhage**.

Risk Factors

The risk factors for placental abruption are:
- Previous placental abruption
- Pre-eclampsia
- Bleeding early in pregnancy
- Trauma (consider domestic violence)
- Multiple pregnancy
- Fetal growth restriction
- Multigravida
- Increased maternal age
- Smoking
- Cocaine or amphetamine use

Presentation

The typical presentation of placental abruption is with:
- Sudden onset severe abdominal pain that is **continuous**
- Vaginal bleeding (antepartum haemorrhage)
- Shock (hypotension and tachycardia)
- Abnormalities on the CTG indicating fetal distress
- Characteristic "**woody**" abdomen on palpation, suggesting a large haemorrhage

Severity of Antepartum Haemorrhage

The RCOG guideline (2011) defines the severity of antepartum haemorrhage as:
- **Spotting**: spots of blood noticed on underwear
- **Minor haemorrhage**: less than 50ml blood loss
- **Major haemorrhage**: 50 - 1000ml blood loss
- **Massive haemorrhage**: more than 1000 ml blood loss, or signs of shock

Concealed Abruption

Concealed abruption is where the **cervical os** remains closed, and any bleeding that occurs remains within the uterine cavity. The severity of bleeding can be significantly underestimated with concealed haemorrhage.

Concealed abruption is opposed to **revealed abruption**, where the blood loss is observed via the vagina.

Management

There are no reliable tests for diagnosing placental abruption. It is a **clinical diagnosis** based on the presentation.

Placental abruption is an obstetric emergency. The urgency depends on the amount of placental separation, extent of bleeding, haemodynamic stability of the mother and condition of the fetus. It is important to consider **concealed haemorrhage**, where the vaginal bleeding may be disproportionate to the uterine bleeding.

The initial steps with major or massive haemorrhage are:
- Urgent involvement of a senior obstetrician, midwife and anaesthetist
- 2 x grey cannula
- Bloods include FBC, UE, LFT and coagulation studies
- Crossmatch 4 units of blood
- Fluid and blood resuscitation as required
- CTG monitoring of the fetus
- Close monitoring of the mother

Ultrasound can be useful in excluding **placenta praevia** as a cause for antepartum haemorrhage, but is not very good at diagnosing or assessing **abruption**.

Antenatal steroids are offered between 24 and 34 + 6 weeks gestation to mature the fetal lungs in anticipation of preterm delivery.

Rhesus-D negative women require **anti-D prophylaxis** when bleeding occurs. A ***Kleihauer test*** is used to quantify how much fetal blood is mixed with the maternal blood, to determine the dose of anti-D that is required.

Emergency caesarean section may be required where the mother is unstable, or there is fetal distress.

There is an increased risk of **postpartum haemorrhage** after delivery in women with placental abruption. ***Active management of the third stage*** is recommended.

Placenta Accreta

Placenta accreta refers to when the placenta implants deeper, through and past the endometrium, making it difficult to separate the placenta after delivery of the baby. It is referred to as **placenta accreta spectrum**, as there is a spectrum of severity in how deep and broad the abnormal implantation extends.

Pathophysiology

There are three layers to the uterine wall:
- **Endometrium**, the **inner layer** that contains connective tissue (**stroma**), **epithelial cells** and **blood vessels**
- **Myometrium**, the **middle layer** that contains **smooth muscle**
- **Perimetrium**, the **outer layer**, which is a **serous membrane** similar to the peritoneum (also known as **serosa**)

Usually the placenta attaches to the **endometrium**. This allows the placenta to separate cleanly during the **third stage of labour**, after delivery of the baby.

With placenta accreta, the placenta embeds past the endometrium, into the myometrium and beyond. This may happen due to a defect in the endometrium. Imperfections may occur due to previous uterine surgery, such as a **caesarean section** or **curettage procedure**. The deep implantation makes it very difficult for the placenta to separate during delivery, leading to extensive bleeding (**postpartum haemorrhage**).

There are three further definitions, depending on the depth of the insertion:
- **Superficial placenta accreta** is where the placenta implants in the surface of the myometrium, but not beyond
- **Placenta increta** is where the placenta attaches deeply into the myometrium
- **Placenta percreta** is where the placenta invades past the myometrium and perimetrium, potentially reaching other organs such as the bladder

Risk Factors

- Previous placenta accreta
- Previous endometrial curettage procedures (e.g. for miscarriage or abortion)
- Previous caesarean section
- Multigravida
- Increased maternal age
- Low-lying placenta or placenta praevia

Presentation

Placenta accreta does not typically cause any symptoms during pregnancy. It can present with bleeding (antepartum haemorrhage) in the third trimester.

It may be diagnosed on **antenatal ultrasound scans**, and particular attention is given during scans to women with a previous placenta accreta or caesarean section to make a diagnosis.

It may be diagnosed at birth, when it becomes difficult to deliver the placenta. It is a cause of significant **postpartum haemorrhage**.

Management

Ideally, placenta accreta is **diagnosed antenatally** by **ultrasound**. This allows planning for birth.

MRI scans may be used to assess the depth and width of the invasion.

A specialist MDT should manage women with placenta accreta. Patients may require additional management at birth due to the risk of bleeding and difficulty separating the placenta. This may include:
- Complex uterine surgery
- Blood transfusions
- Intensive care for the mother
- Neonatal intensive care

Delivery is planned between 35 to 36 + 6 weeks gestation to reduce the risk of spontaneous labour and delivery. Antenatal steroids are given to mature the fetal lungs before delivery.

The options during caesarean are:
- **Hysterectomy** with the placenta remaining in the uterus (recommended)
- **Uterus preserving surgery**, with resection of part of the myometrium along with the placenta
- **Expectant management**, leaving the placenta in place to be reabsorbed over time

Expectant management comes with significant risks, particularly bleeding and infection.

The RCOG guideline (2018) suggests that if placenta accreta is seen when opening the abdomen for an elective caesarean section, the abdomen can be closed and delivery delayed whilst specialist services are put in place. If placenta accreta is discovered after delivery of the baby, a hysterectomy is recommended.

Breech Presentation

Breech presentation refers to when the presenting part of the fetus (the lowest part) is the legs and bottom. This is opposed to **cephalic presentation**, where the head is the presenting part. Breech presentation occurs in less than 5% of pregnancies by 37 weeks gestation.

Types of Breech

- **Complete breech**, where the legs are fully flexed at the hips and knees
- **Incomplete breech**, with one leg flexed at the hip and extended at the knee

- **Extended breech**, also known as frank breech, with both legs flexed at the hip and extended at the knee
- **Footling breech**, when a foot is presenting through the cervix, with the leg extended

Management

Babies that are breech before 36 weeks often turn spontaneously, so no intervention is advised. **External cephalic version** (**ECV**) can be used at term (37 weeks) to attempt to turn the fetus.

Where ECV fails, women are given a choice between **vaginal delivery** and **elective caesarean section**. Vaginal delivery needs to involve experienced midwives and obstetricians, with access to emergency theatre if required.

Overall, vaginal birth is safer for the mother, and caesarean section is safer for the baby. There is about a 40% chance of requiring an emergency caesarean section when vaginal birth is attempted.

When the first baby in a twin pregnancy is breech, caesarean section is required.

External Cephalic Version

External cephalic version (**ECV**) is a technique used to attempt to turn a fetus from the breech position to a cephalic position using pressure on the pregnant abdomen. It is about 50% successful.

External cephalic version is used in babies that are breech:
- After 36 weeks for nulliparous women (women that have not previously given birth)
- After 37 weeks in women that have given birth previously

Women are given **tocolysis** to relax the uterus before the procedure. Tocolysis is with **subcutaneous terbutaline**. Terbutaline is a **beta-agonist** similar to salbutamol. It reduces the **contractility** of the **myometrium**, making it easier for the baby to turn.

Rhesus-D negative women require **anti-D prophylaxis** when ECV is performed. A **Kleihauer test** is used to quantify how much fetal blood is mixed with the maternal blood, to determine the dose of anti-D that is required.

Stillbirth

Stillbirth is defined as the birth of a dead fetus after 24 weeks gestation. Stillbirth is the result of **intrauterine fetal death** (**IUFD**). It occurs in approximately 1 in 200 pregnancies.

Causes

Many of the conditions that can affect pregnancy increase the risk of stillbirth. Unexplained stillbirth is common. The causes of stillbirth include:

- Unexplained (around 50%)
- Pre-eclampsia
- Placental abruption
- Vasa praevia
- Cord prolapse or wrapped around the fetal neck
- Obstetric cholestasis
- Diabetes
- Thyroid disease
- Infections, such as rubella, parvovirus and listeria
- Genetic abnormalities or congenital malformations

Factors that increase the risk of stillbirth include:
- Fetal growth restriction
- Smoking
- Alcohol
- Increased maternal age
- Maternal obesity
- Twins
- Sleeping on the back (as opposed to either side)

Prevention

A risk assessment for having a baby that is **small for gestational age** (**SGA**) or with **fetal growth restriction** (**FGR**) is performed on all pregnant women. Having risk factors for SGA increases the risk of stillbirth. Those at risk have the fetal growth closely monitored with **serial growth scans**. This helps identify women that need further investigations and management. They may need planned early delivery when the growth is static, or other concerns are identified.

Women at risk of **pre-eclampsia** are given **aspirin**. Any modifiable risk factors for stillbirth are treated, for example, stopping smoking, avoiding alcohol and effective control of diabetes. Sleeping on the side (not the back) is advised.

There are three key symptoms to always ask about during pregnancy. Women would report these immediately if they occur:
- Reduced fetal movements
- Abdominal pain
- Vaginal bleeding

Management

Ultrasound scan is the investigation of choice for diagnosing **intrauterine fetal death** (**IUFD**). It is used to visualise the **fetal heartbeat** to confirm the fetus is still alive.

Passive fetal movements are possible after IUFD, and a repeat scan is offered to confirm the situation.

Rhesus-D negative women require **anti-D prophylaxis** when IUFD is diagnosed. A **Kleihauer test** is used to quantify how much fetal blood is mixed with the maternal blood, to determine the dose of anti-D that is required.

Vaginal birth is first-line for most women after IUFD, unless there are other reasons for caesarean section. Women are given a choice of **induction of labour** or **expectant management** (provided immediate delivery is not required, for example with sepsis, pre-eclampsia or haemorrhage). **Expectant management** involves awaiting natural labour and delivery. Women with expectant management need close monitoring. The condition of the fetus will deteriorate with time.

Induction of labour involves using a combination of oral **mifepristone** (**anti-progesterone**) and vaginal or oral **misoprostol** (**prostaglandin analogue**).

Dopamine agonists (e.g. **cabergoline**) can be used to **suppress lactation** after stillbirth.

With **parental consent**, testing is carried out after stillbirth to determine the cause:
- Genetic testing of the fetus and placenta
- Postmortem examination of the fetus (including xrays)
- Testing for maternal and fetal infection
- Testing the mother for conditions associated with stillbirth, such as diabetes, thyroid disease and thrombophilia

Identifying the cause can help reduce the risk in future pregnancies. Pregnancies are closely monitored in women with previous stillbirth.

Sensitive **breaking bad news** and good **emotional support** is essential, provided in an appropriate place by appropriately trained and experienced staff. Counselling is offered to women, partners and family members. They are supported with their individual wishes, such as seeing the baby, naming the baby and keeping photographs (although not persuaded either way with what to do). They are also supported with wishes for funeral arrangements and services.

Cardiac Arrest in Pregnancy

There are differences between cardiac arrest and resuscitation in pregnancy compared with standard adult resuscitation. Always follow local and national guidelines, get formal training and involve experienced seniors when managing critically ill patients. The relevant RCOG guidelines on maternal collapse are from 2011. This overview is to help you understand the concepts in preparation for your exams.

Causes of Cardiac Arrest in Pregnancy

The Resuscitation Council UK list the **reversible causes** of adult cardiac arrest as the **4 Ts** and **4 Hs**:

- **Thrombosis** (i.e. PE or MI)
- **Tension pneumothorax**
- **Toxins**
- **Tamponade** (cardiac)

- **Hypoxia**
- **Hypovolaemia**
- **Hypothermia**
- **Hyperkalaemia**, **hypoglycaemia**, and other **metabolic abnormalities**

The RCOG guideline advises adding to the list:

- **Eclampsia**
- **Intracranial haemorrhage**

The three major causes of cardiac arrest in pregnancy to remember are:
- **Obstetric haemorrhage**
- **Pulmonary embolism**
- **Sepsis** leading to **metabolic acidosis** and **septic shock**

Obstetric haemorrhage is a major cause of severe **hypovolaemia** and cardiac arrest. Remember the causes of massive obstetric haemorrhage:
- **Ectopic pregnancy** (early pregnancy)
- **Placental abruption** (including **concealed haemorrhage**)
- **Placenta praevia**
- **Placenta accreta**
- **Uterine rupture**

Aortocaval Compression

After 20 weeks gestation, the uterus is a significant size. When a pregnant woman lies on her back (**supine**), the mass of the uterus can compress the **inferior vena cava** and **aorta**. The compression on the **vena cava** is most significant, as it reduces the blood return to the heart (**venous return**). This reduces the **cardiac output**, leading to **hypotension**. In some instances, this can be enough to lead to the loss of **cardiac output** and **cardiac arrest**.

The vena cava is slightly to the right side of the body. The solution to aortocaval compression is to place the woman in the **left lateral position**, lying on her left side, with the pregnant uterus positioned away from the inferior vena cava. This should relieve the compression on the inferior vena cava and improve venous return and cardiac output.

Resuscitation in Pregnancy

Several factors make resuscitation more complicated in pregnancy:
- Aortocaval compression
- Increased oxygen requirements
- Splinting of the diaphragm by the pregnant abdomen
- Difficulty with intubation
- Increased risk of aspiration
- Ongoing obstetric haemorrhage

Resuscitation in pregnancy follows the same principles as standard adult life support, except for:
- A **15 degree tilt** to the **left side** for CPR, to relieve compression of the inferior vena cava and aorta
- Early intubation to protect the airway
- Early supplementary oxygen
- Aggressive fluid resuscitation (caution in pre-eclampsia)
- Delivery of the baby after 4 minutes, and within 5 minutes of starting CPR

Delivery

Immediate caesarean section is performed in a pregnant woman when:
- There is no response after 4 minutes to CPR performed correctly
- CPR continues for more than 4 minutes in a woman more than 20 weeks gestation

The aim is to deliver the baby and placenta within 5 minutes of CPR commencing. The operation is performed at the site of the arrest, for example, in A&E resus or on the ward.

The primary reason for the immediate delivery is to **improve the survival of the mother**. Delivery improves the venous return to the heart, improves cardiac output and reduces oxygen consumption. It also helps with ventilation and chest compressions. Delivery increases the chances of the baby surviving, although this is secondary to the survival of the mother.

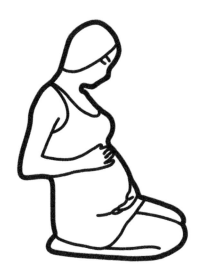

LABOUR AND DELIVERY

9.1	The Onset of Labour	192
9.2	Premature Labour	193
9.3	Induction of Labour	195
9.4	Cardiotocography	197
9.5	Drugs in Labour	200
9.6	Failure to Progress	202
9.7	Pain Relief in Labour	205
9.8	Umbilical Cord Prolapse	206
9.9	Shoulder Dystocia	207
9.10	Instrumental Delivery	208
9.11	Perineal Tears	209
9.12	Active Management of the Third Stage	211
9.13	Postpartum Haemorrhage	212
9.14	Caesarean Section	214
9.15	Maternal Sepsis	217
9.16	Amniotic Fluid Embolisation	219
9.17	Uterine Rupture	220
9.18	Uterine Inversion	221

The Onset of Labour

Labour and delivery normally occur between 37 and 42 weeks gestation.

There are three stages of labour:
- *First stage* - from the onset of labour (true contractions) until 10cm cervical dilatation
- *Second stage* - from 10cm cervical dilatation until delivery of the baby
- *Third stage* - from delivery of the baby until delivery of the placenta

First Stage

The first stage of labour is from the onset of labour (true contractions) until the cervix is fully dilated to 10cm. It involves **cervical dilation** (opening up) and **effacement** (getting thinner). The "**show**" refers to the **mucus plug** in the cervix, which prevents bacteria from entering the uterus during pregnancy, falling out and creating space for the baby to pass through.

The first stage has three **phases**:
- *Latent phase* - from 0 to 3cm dilation of the cervix. This progresses at around 0.5cm per hour. There are irregular contractions.
- *Active phase* - from 3cm to 7cm dilation of the cervix. This progresses at around 1cm per hour, and there are regular contractions.
- *Transition phase* - from 7cm to 10cm dilation of the cervix. This progresses at around 1cm per hour, and there are strong and regular contractions.

Braxton-Hicks Contractions

Braxton-Hicks contractions are occasional irregular contractions of the uterus. They are usually felt during the second and third trimester. Women can experience temporary and irregular tightening or mild cramping in the abdomen. These are not true contractions, and they **do not** indicate the onset of labour. They do not progress or become regular. Staying hydrated and relaxing can help reduce Braxton-Hicks contractions.

Diagnosing the Onset of Labour

The signs of labour are:
- *Show* (mucus plug from the cervix)
- *Rupture of membranes*
- *Regular, painful* contractions
- *Dilating cervix* on examination

NICE guidelines on intrapartum care (2017) refer to the *latent first stage* and *established first stage*.

The *latent first stage* is when there are both:
- Painful contractions
- Changes to the cervix, with effacement and dilation up to 4cm

The *established first stage* is when there are both:
- Regular, painful contractions
- Dilatation of the cervix from 4cm onwards

Premature Labour

Definitions

***Rupture of membranes** (**ROM**)*: The amniotic sac has ruptured.

***Spontaneous rupture of membranes** (**SROM**)*: The amniotic sac has ruptured spontaneously.

***Prelabour rupture of membranes** (**PROM**)*: The amniotic sac has ruptured before the onset of labour.

***Preterm prelabour rupture of membranes** (**P-PROM**)*: The amniotic sac has ruptured before the onset of labour and before 37 weeks gestation (preterm).

***Prolonged rupture of membranes** (**also PROM**)*: The amniotic sac ruptures more than 18 hours before delivery.

Prematurity

Prematurity is defined as birth before **37 weeks gestation**. The more premature the baby, the worse the outcomes.

Babies are considered **non-viable** below 23 weeks gestation. Generally, from 23 to 24 weeks, resuscitation is not considered in babies that do not show signs of life. Babies born at 23 weeks have around a 10% chance of survival. From 24 weeks onwards, there is an increased chance of survival, and full resuscitation is offered.

The World Health Organisation classify prematurity as:
- Under 28 weeks: **extreme preterm**
- 28 – 32 weeks: **very preterm**
- 32 – 37 weeks: **moderate to late preterm**

Prophylaxis of Preterm Labour

Vaginal Progesterone

Progesterone can be given vaginally via a gel or pessary as prophylaxis for preterm labour. Progesterone has a role in maintaining pregnancy and preventing labour by decreasing activity of the myometrium and preventing the cervix remodelling in preparation for delivery. This is offered to women with a cervical length less than 25mm on vaginal ultrasound between 16 and 24 weeks gestation.

Cervical Cerclage

Cervical cerclage involves putting a stitch in the cervix to add support and keep it closed. This involves a spinal or general anaesthetic. The stitch is removed when the woman goes into labour or reaches term.

Cervical cerclage is offered to women with a cervical length less than 25mm on vaginal ultrasound between 16 and 24 weeks gestation, who have had a previous premature birth or cervical trauma (e.g. colposcopy and cone biopsy).

"**Rescue**" cervical cerclage may also be offered between 16 and 27 + 6 weeks when there is cervical dilatation without rupture of membranes, to prevent progression and premature delivery.

Preterm Prelabour Rupture of Membranes

Preterm prelabour rupture of membranes is where the **amniotic sac** ruptures, releasing **amniotic fluid**, before the onset of labour and in a preterm pregnancy (under 37 weeks gestation).

Diagnosis

Rupture of membranes can be diagnosed by speculum examination revealing pooling of amniotic fluid in the vagina. No tests are required.

Where there is doubt about the diagnosis, tests can be performed:
- **Insulin-like growth factor-binding protein-1** (**IGFBP-1**) is a protein present in high concentrations in amniotic fluid, which can be tested on vaginal fluid if there is doubt about rupture of membranes
- **Placental alpha-microglobin-1** (**PAMG-1**) is a similar alternative to IGFBP-1

Management

Prophylactic antibiotics should be given to prevent the development of **chorioamnionitis**. The NICE guidelines (2019) recommend erythromycin 250mg four times daily for ten days, or until labour is established if within ten days.

Induction of labour may be offered from 34 weeks to initiate the onset of labour.

Preterm Labour with Intact Membranes

Preterm labour with intact membranes involves regular painful contractions and cervical dilatation, without rupture of the amniotic sac.

Diagnosis

Clinical assessment includes a speculum examination to assess for cervical dilatation. The NICE guidelines (2017) recommend:
- Less than **30 weeks gestation**, clinical assessment alone is enough to offer management of preterm labour.
- More than **30 weeks gestation**, a **transvaginal ultrasound** can be used to assess the **cervical length**. When the cervical length on ultrasound is less than 15mm, management of preterm labour can be offered. A cervical length of more than 15mm indicates preterm labour is unlikely.

Fetal fibronectin is an alternative test to vaginal ultrasound. Fetal fibronectin is the "glue" between the chorion and the uterus, and is found in the vagina during labour. A result of less than 50 ng/ml is considered negative, and indicates that preterm labour is unlikely.

Management

There are several options for improving the outcomes in preterm labour:
- **Fetal monitoring** (CTG or intermittent auscultation)
- **Tocolysis with nifedipine**: nifedipine is a calcium channel blocker that suppresses labour
- **Maternal corticosteroids**: can be offered before 35 weeks gestation to reduce neonatal morbidity and mortality
- **IV magnesium sulphate**: can be given before 34 weeks gestation and helps protect the baby's brain
- **Delayed cord clamping** or **cord milking**: can increase the circulating blood volume and haemoglobin in the baby at birth

Tocolysis

Tocolysis involves using medications to stop uterine contractions. **Nifedipine**, a calcium channel blocker, is the medication of choice for tocolysis. **Atosiban** is an **oxytocin receptor antagonist** that can be used as an alternative when nifedipine is contraindicated.

Tocolysis can be used between 24 and 33 + 6 weeks gestation in preterm labour to delay delivery and buy time for further fetal development, administration of maternal steroids or transfer to a more specialist unit (e.g. with a neonatal ICU). It is only used as a short-term measure (i.e. less than 48 hours).

Antenatal Steroids

Giving the mother **corticosteroids** helps to develop the fetal lungs and reduce **respiratory distress syndrome** after delivery. They are used in women with suspected preterm labour *less than 36 weeks gestation*.

An example regime would be **two doses** of **intramuscular betamethasone**, 24 hours apart.

Magnesium Sulfate

Giving the mother **IV magnesium sulfate** helps protect the **fetal brain** during premature delivery. It reduces the risk and severity of **cerebral palsy**. Magnesium sulfate is given within 24 hours of **delivery** of preterm babies of *less than 34 weeks gestation*. It is given as a bolus, followed by an infusion for up to 24 hours or until birth.

Mothers need close monitoring for **magnesium toxicity** at least four hourly. This involves close monitoring of observations, as well as **tendon reflexes** (usually **patella reflex**). Key signs of toxicity are:
- Reduced respiratory rate
- Reduced blood pressure
- Absent reflexes

Induction of Labour

Induction of labour (IOL) refers to the use of medications to stimulate the onset of labour.

Indications

Induction of labour can be used where patients go over the due date. IOL is offered between 41 and 42 weeks gestation.

Induction of labour is also offered in situations where it is beneficial to start labour early, such as:
- Prelabour rupture of membranes
- Fetal growth restriction
- Pre-eclampsia
- Obstetric cholestasis
- Existing diabetes
- Intrauterine fetal death

Bishop Score

The Bishop score is a scoring system used to determine whether to proceed with induction of labour.

Five things are assessed and given a score based on different criteria (minimum score is 0 and maximum is 13):
- Fetal station (scored 0 - 3)
- Cervical position (scored 0 - 2)
- Cervical dilatation (scored 0 - 3)
- Cervical effacement (scored 0 - 3)
- Cervical consistency (scored 0 - 2)

A score of 8 or more predicts a successful induction of labour. A score below this suggests cervical ripening may be required to prepare the cervix before induction.

Options for Induction of Labour

Membrane sweep involves inserting a finger into the cervix to stimulate the cervix and begin the process of labour. It can be performed in antenatal clinic, and if successful, should produce the onset of labour within 48 hours. A membrane sweep is not considered a full method of inducing labour, and is more of an assistance before full induction of labour. It is used from 40 weeks gestation to attempt to initiate labour in women over their EDD.

Vaginal prostaglandin E2 (**dinoprostone**) involves inserting a **gel**, **tablet** (**Prostin**) or **pessary** (**Propess**) into the vagina. The pessary is similar to a tampon, and slowly releases local **prostaglandins** over 24 hours. This stimulates the cervix and uterus to cause the onset of labour. This is usually done in the hospital setting so that the woman can be monitored before being allowed home to await the full onset of labour.

Cervical ripening balloon (**CRB**) is a silicone balloon that is inserted into the cervix and gently inflated to dilate the cervix. This is used as an alternative where vaginal prostaglandins are not preferred, usually in women with a previous caesarean section, where vaginal prostaglandins have failed or multiparous women (para ≥ 3).

Artificial rupture of membranes with an **oxytocin infusion** can also be used to induce labour, although this would only be used where there are reasons not to use vaginal prostaglandins. It can be used to progress the induction of labour after vaginal prostaglandins have already initiated the process.

Oral mifepristone (**anti-progesterone**) plus **misoprostol** are used to induce labour where **intrauterine fetal death** has occurred.

Monitoring

There are two means for monitoring during the induction of labour.
- **Cardiotocography** (**CTG**) to assess the fetal heart rate and uterine contractions before and during induction of labour
- **Bishop score** before and during induction of labour to monitor the progress

Ongoing Management

Most women will give birth within 24 hours of the start of induction of labour. The options when there is slow or no progress are:
- Further vaginal prostaglandins
- Artificial rupture of membranes and oxytocin infusion
- Cervical ripening balloon (CRB)
- Elective caesarean section

Uterine Hyperstimulation

Uterine hyperstimulation is the main complication of induction of labour with vaginal prostaglandins. This is where the contraction of the uterus is prolonged and frequent, causing fetal distress and compromise.

The criteria for uterine hyperstimulation varies slightly between guidelines (always check local policies and involve experienced seniors). The two criteria often given are:
- Individual uterine contractions lasting more than 2 minutes in duration
- More than five uterine contractions every 10 minutes

Uterine hyperstimulation can lead to:
- Fetal compromise, with hypoxia and acidosis
- Emergency caesarean section
- Uterine rupture

Management of uterine hyperstimulation involves:
- Removing the vaginal prostaglandins, or stopping the oxytocin infusion
- **Tocolysis** with **terbutaline**

Cardiotocography

Cardiotocography (**CTG**) is used to measure the **fetal heart rate** and the **contractions of the uterus**. It is also known as **electronic fetal monitoring**. It is a useful way of monitoring the condition of the fetus and the activity of labour.

CTG can help guide decision making and delivery. However, it should not be used in isolation for decision making, and it is essential to take into account the overall clinical picture.

Operation

Two transducers are placed on the abdomen to get the CTG readout:
- One above the fetal heart to monitor the fetal heartbeat
- One near the fundus of the uterus to monitor the uterine contractions

The transducer above the fetal heart monitors the heartbeat using **Doppler ultrasound**. The transducer above the fundus uses ultrasound to assess the **tension** in the uterine wall, demonstrating **uterine contractions**.

Indications for Continuous CTG Monitoring

The indications for **continuous CTG** monitoring in labour include:
- Sepsis
- Maternal tachycardia (> 120)
- Significant meconium
- Pre-eclampsia (particularly blood pressure > 160 / 110)
- Fresh antepartum haemorrhage
- Delay in labour
- Use of oxytocin
- Disproportionate maternal pain

Key Features

There are five key features to look for on a CTG:
- **Contractions** - the number of uterine contractions per 10 minutes
- **Baseline rate** - the baseline fetal heart rate
- **Variability** - how the fetal heart rate varies up and down around the baseline
- **Accelerations** - periods where the fetal heart rate spikes
- **Decelerations** - periods where the fetal heart rate drops

Contractions

Contractions are used to gauge the activity of labour. Too few contractions indicate labour is not progressing. Too many contractions can mean **uterine hyperstimulation**, which can lead to fetal compromise. It is also important to interpret the fetal heart rate in the context of the uterine contractions.

Accelerations

Accelerations are generally a good sign that the fetus is healthy, particularly when occurring alongside contraction of the uterus.

Baseline Rate and Variability

Baseline rate and variability can be described as **reassuring**, **non-reassuring** and **abnormal** (adapted from NICE guidelines 2017):

Feature	Reassuring	Non-reassuring	Abnormal
Baseline rate	110 - 160	100 - 109 or 161 - 180	Below 100 or above 180
Variability	5 - 25	Less than 5 for 30 - 50 minutes or More than 25 for 15 - 25 minutes	Less than 5 for over 50 minutes or More than 25 for over 25 minutes

Decelerations

Decelerations are a more concerning finding. The fetal heart rate drops in response to **hypoxia**. The fetal heart rate is slowing to conserve oxygen for the vital organs. There are four types of decelerations to be aware of:
- **Early decelerations**
- **Late decelerations**
- **Variable decelerations**
- **Prolonged decelerations**

Early decelerations are gradual dips and recoveries in heart rate that correspond with uterine contractions. The lowest point of the deceleration corresponds to the peak of the contraction. Early decelerations are normal and not considered pathological. They are caused by the uterus compressing the head the fetus, stimulating the **vagus nerve**, causing the heart rate to slow.

Late decelerations are gradual falls in heart rate that starts **after** the uterine contraction has already begun. There is a delay between the uterine contraction and the deceleration. The lowest point of the deceleration occurs **after** the peak of the contraction. Late decelerations are caused by **hypoxia** in the fetus, and are a more concerning finding. They may be caused by excessive uterine contractions, maternal hypotension or maternal hypoxia.

Variable decelerations are abrupt decelerations that may be unrelated to uterine contractions. There is a fall of more than 15 bpm from the baseline. The lowest point of the deceleration occurs within 30 seconds, and the deceleration lasts less than 2 minutes in total. Variable decelerations often indicate intermittent compression of the umbilical cord, causing fetal hypoxia. Brief **accelerations** before and after the deceleration are known as **shoulders**, and are a reassuring sign that the fetus is coping.

Prolonged decelerations last between 2 and 10 minutes, with a drop of more than 15 bpm from baseline. This often indicates compression of the umbilical cord, causing fetal hypoxia. These are abnormal and concerning.

The NICE guidelines (2017) have criteria for describing findings of decelerations as **reassuring**, **non-reassuring** and **abnormal**. It is worth remembering that the CTG is **reassuring** when there are **no decelerations**, **early decelerations** or less than 90 minutes of **variable decelerations** with no concerning features.

Regular variable decelerations and late decelerations are classed as non-reassuring or abnormal, depending on the features. Prolonged decelerations are always abnormal.

Management Based on the CTG

The NICE guidelines (2017) recommend categorising the CTG based on three features of the CTG described above:
- Baseline rate
- Variability
- Decelerations

The four categories for CTG are:
- **Normal**
- **Suspicious**: a single non-reassuring feature
- **Pathological**: two non-reassuring features or a single abnormal feature
- **Need for urgent intervention**: acute bradycardia or prolonged deceleration of more than 3 minutes

The outcome of the CTG will guide management, such as:
- **Escalating** to a senior midwife and obstetrician
- **Further assessment** for possible causes, such as uterine hyperstimulation, maternal hypotension and cord prolapse
- **Conservative interventions** such as repositioning the mother or giving IV fluids for hypotension
- **Fetal scalp stimulation** (an acceleration in response to stimulation is a reassuring sign)
- **Fetal scalp blood sampling** to test for fetal acidosis
- **Delivery of the baby** (e.g. instrumental delivery or emergency caesarean section)

Fetal Bradycardia

There is a "rule of 3's" for fetal bradycardia when they are prolonged:
- 3 minutes - call for help
- 6 minutes - move to theatre
- 9 minutes - prepare for delivery
- 12 minutes - deliver the baby (by 15 minutes)

Sinusoidal CTG

A sinusoidal CTG is a rare pattern to be aware of, as it can indicate severe fetal compromise. It gives a pattern similar to a **sine wave**, with smooth regular waves up and down that have an amplitude of 5 - 15 bpm. It is usually associated with severe fetal anaemia, for example, caused by vasa praevia with fetal haemorrhage.

DR C BRaVADO

DR C BRaVADO is a mnemonic often taught to assess the features of a CTG in a structured way. It involves assessing in order:
- **DR** - **D**efine **R**isk (define the risk based on the individual woman and pregnancy before assessing the CTG)
- **C** - **C**ontractions
- **BRa** - **B**aseline **Ra**te
- **V** - **V**ariability
- **A** - **A**ccelerations
- **D** - **D**ecelerations
- **O** - **O**verall impression (give an overall impression of the CTG and clinical picture)

If you are asked to assess a CTG in your exams, use the DR C BRaVADO structure to describe each feature in turn. Give an overall impression of the CTG as being **normal** (all features are reassuring), **suspicious**, **pathological**, or **need for urgent intervention**, as described in the NICE guidelines (2017).

Drugs in Labour

There are numerous medications that may be used during labour. This section includes the main ones to clarify what they are, how they work and when they are used.

Oxytocin

Oxytocin is a hormone secreted by the **posterior pituitary gland**. It is produced in the **hypothalamus**, but travels to the pituitary before being released into the general circulation. It has several effects on mood and social interactions in everyday life, but also plays a vital role in labour and delivery.

Oxytocin stimulates the **ripening of the cervix** and **contractions of the uterus** during labour and delivery. It also plays a role in **lactation** during **breastfeeding**.

Infusions of oxytocin are used to:
- Induce labour
- Progress labour
- Improve the frequency and strength of uterine contractions
- Prevent or treat postpartum haemorrhage

Syntocinon is a brand name for oxytocin produced by one drug company.

Atosiban is an **oxytocin receptor antagonist** that can be used as an alternative to nifedipine for **tocolysis** in premature labour (when nifedipine is contraindicated).

Ergometrine

Ergometrine is derived from **ergot plants**. It stimulates smooth muscle contraction, both in the uterus and blood vessels. This makes it useful for delivery of the placenta and to reduce postpartum bleeding. It may be used during the **third stage** of labour (delivery of the placenta) and **postpartum** to prevent and treat **postpartum haemorrhage**. It is only used **after** delivery of the baby, not in the first or second stage.

Due to the action on the smooth muscle in blood vessels and gastrointestinal tract, it can cause several side effects, including **hypertension**, **diarrhoea**, **vomiting** and **angina**. It needs to be avoided in eclampsia, and used only with significant caution in patients with hypertension.

Syntometrine is a combination drug containing **oxytocin** (Syntocinon) and **ergometrine**. It can be used for prevention or treatment of postpartum haemorrhage.

Prostaglandins

Prostaglandins act like local hormones, triggering specific effects in local tissues. Tissues throughout the entire body contain and respond to prostaglandins. They play a crucial role in menstruation and labour by stimulating contraction of the uterine muscles. They also have a role in ripening the cervix before delivery.

One key prostaglandin to be aware of is **dinoprostone**, which is **prostaglandin E2**. This is used for induction of labour, and can come in one of three forms:
- Vaginal **pessaries** (**Propess**)
- Vaginal **tablets** (**Prostin** tablets)
- Vaginal **gel** (**Prostin gel**)

TOM TIP: Prostaglandins act as vasodilators, and lower blood pressure. NSAIDs such as ibuprofen and naproxen inhibit the action of prostaglandins. As a result, NSAIDs can increase blood pressure. NSAIDs are generally avoided in pregnancy, and also after delivery in women with raised blood pressure (although research has shed doubt on whether the effect on blood pressure is significant enough to justify avoiding them). NSAIDs (e.g. ibuprofen and mefenamic acid) are useful in treating dysmenorrhoea (painful periods), as they reduce the painful cramping of the uterus during menstruation.

Misoprostol

Misoprostol is a **prostaglandin analogue**, meaning it binds to **prostaglandin receptors** and activates them. It is used as medical management in miscarriage, to help complete the miscarriage. Misoprostol is used alongside **mifepristone** for **abortions**, and **induction of labour** after **intrauterine fetal death**.

Mifepristone

Mifepristone is an **anti-progestogen** medication that blocks the action of **progesterone**, halting the pregnancy and ripening the cervix. It enhances the effects of prostaglandins to stimulate contraction of the uterus. Mifepristone is used alongside **misoprostol** for **abortions**, and **induction of labour** after **intrauterine fetal death**. It is not used during pregnancy with a healthy living fetus.

Nifedipine

Nifedipine is a **calcium channel blocker** that acts to reduce **smooth muscle contraction** in **blood vessels** and the **uterus**. It has two main uses in pregnancy:
- **Reduce blood pressure** in hypertension and pre-eclampsia
- **Tocolysis** in premature labour, where it suppresses uterine activity and delays the onset of labour

Terbutaline

Terbutaline is a **beta-2 agonist**, similar to salbutamol. It stimulates **beta-2 adrenergic receptors**. It acts on the smooth muscle of the uterus to suppress uterine contractions. It is used for **tocolysis** in **uterine hyperstimulation**, notably when the uterine contractions become excessive during **induction of labour**.

Carboprost

Carboprost is a **synthetic prostaglandin analogue**, meaning it binds to **prostaglandin receptors**. It stimulates uterine contraction. It is given as a **deep intramuscular injection** in **postpartum haemorrhage**, where ergometrine and oxytocin have been inadequate. Notably, it needs to be avoided, or used with particular caution, in patients with asthma, as it can cause a potentially life-threatening exacerbation of the asthma.

Tranexamic Acid

Tranexamic acid is an **antifibrinolytic** that reduces bleeding. It binds to **fibrinogen** and prevents it from converting to **plasmin**. **Plasmin** is an **enzyme** the helps break down **fibrin blood clots**. Therefore, tranexamic acid helps prevent the breakdown of blood clots. It also **inhibits** the action of **fibrin**, a protein involved in the formation of blood clots.

Tranexamic acid is used in the prevention and treatment of **postpartum haemorrhage**.

Failure to Progress

Failure to progress refers to when labour is not developing at a satisfactory rate. This increases the risk to the fetus and the mother. It is more likely to occur in women in labour for the first time compared with those that have previously given birth.

Progress in labour is influenced by the three P's:
- **Power** (uterine contractions)
- **Passenger** (size, presentation and position of the baby)
- **Passage** (the shape and size of the pelvis and soft tissues)

Psyche can be added as a fourth P, referring to the support and antenatal preparation for labour and delivery.

First Stage of Labour

The first stage has three **phases**:
- **Latent phase** - from 0 to 3cm dilation of the cervix. This progresses at around 0.5cm per hour. There are irregular contractions.

- **Active phase** - from 3cm to 7cm dilation of the cervix. This progresses at around 1cm per hour, and there are regular contractions.
- **Transition phase** - from 7cm to 10cm dilation of the cervix. This progresses at around 1cm per hour, and there are strong and regular contractions.

Delay in the first stage of labour is considered when there is either:
- Less than 2cm of cervical dilatation in 4 hours
- Slowing of progress in a multiparous women

Partogram

Women are monitored for their progress in the **first stage** of labour using a **partogram**. It is worth becoming familiar with partograms and how they are recorded.

Recorded on a partogram are:
- **Cervical dilatation** (measured by a 4-hourly vaginal examination)
- **Descent of the fetal head** (in relation to the **ischial spines**)
- Maternal pulse, blood pressure, temperature and urine output
- Fetal heart rate
- Frequency of contractions
- Status of the membranes, presence of liquor and whether the liquor is stained by blood or meconium
- Drugs and fluids that have been given

Uterine contractions are measure in contractions per 10 minutes. When the midwife says "she is contracting 2 in 10", it means she is having 2 uterine contractions in a 10 minute period.

There are two lines on the partogram that indicate when labour may not be progressing adequately. These are labelled "*alert*" and "*action*". The dilation of the cervix is plotted against the duration of labour (time). When it takes too long for the cervix to dilate, the readings will cross to the right of the *alert* and *action* lines.

Crossing the *alert line* is an indication for **amniotomy** (artificially rupturing the membranes) and a repeat examination in 2 hours. Crossing the action line means care needs to be escalated to **obstetric-led care** and senior decision-makers for appropriate action.

Second Stage

The second stage of labour lasts from 10cm dilatation of the cervix to delivery of the baby. The success of the second stage depends on "**the three Ps**": **power**, **passenger** and **passage**. **Delay in the second stage** is when it lasts over:
- 2 hours in a nulliparous woman
- 1 hour in a multiparous woman

Power
Power refers to the strength of the uterine contractions. When there are weak uterine contractions, an oxytocin infusion can be used to stimulate the uterus.

Passenger
Passenger refers to the four descriptive qualities of the fetus:
- Size
- Attitude
- Lie
- Presentation

Size refers to the size of the baby. Large babies (macrosomia) will be more difficult to deliver, and there may be issues such as **shoulder dystocia**. The size of the head is important as this is the largest part of the fetus.

Attitude refers to the posture of the fetus. For example, how the back is rounded and how the head and limbs are flexed.

Lie refers to the position of the fetus in relation to the mother's body:
- Longitudinal lie - the fetus is straight up and down
- Transverse lie - the fetus is straight side to side
- Oblique lie - the fetus is at an angle

Presentation refers to the part of the fetus closest to the cervix:
- Cephalic presentation - the head is first
- Shoulder presentation - the shoulder is first
- Breech presentation - the legs are first. This can be:
  - Complete breech - with hips and knees flexed (like doing a cannonball jump into a pool)
  - Frank breech - with hips flexed and knees extended, bottom first
  - Footling breech - with a foot hanging through the cervix

Passage: the size and shape of the passageway, mainly the pelvis.

When there are problems in the second stage of labour, interventions may be required depending on the situation. Possible interventions include:
- Changing positions
- Encouragement
- Analgesia
- Oxytocin
- Episiotomy
- Instrumental delivery
- Caesarean section

Third Stage

The third stage of labour is from delivery of the baby to delivery of the placenta. Delay in the third stage is defined by the NICE guidelines (2017) as:
- More than 30 minutes with active management
- More than 60 minutes with physiological management

Active management involves **intramuscular oxytocin** and **controlled cord traction**.

Management of Failure to Progress

Experienced midwives and obstetricians will manage failure to progress. The main options for managing failure to progress are:
- **Amniotomy**, also known as **artificial rupture of membranes** (**ARM**) for women with intact membranes
- **Oxytocin infusion**
- **Instrumental delivery**
- **Caesarean section**

Oxytocin is used first-line to stimulate uterine contractions during labour. It is started at a low rate and titrated up at intervals of at least 30 minutes as required. The aim is for 4 - 5 contractions per 10 minutes. Too few contractions will mean that labour does not progress. Too many contractions can result in fetal compromise, as the fetus does not have the opportunity to recover between contractions.

The condition of the fetus needs to be monitored throughout labour and delivery. Fetal compromise may mean delivery needs to be expedited, or example, with emergency caesarean section.

Pain Relief in Labour

There are several options for pain relief in labour. This section covers the main medical options.

Antenatal classes help prepare women for what to expect in labour, and can make the experience more comfortable and less scary. Several things can improve the symptoms without medications:
- Understanding what to expect
- Having good support
- Being in a relaxed environment
- Changing position to stay comfortable
- Controlled breathing
- Water births may help some women
- TENS machines may be useful in the early stages of labour

Simple Analgesia

Paracetamol is frequently used in early labour. Codeine may be added for additional effect. NSAIDs are avoided.

Gas and Air (Entonox)

Gas and air contains a mixture of 50% **nitrous oxide** and 50% **oxygen**. This is used during contractions for short term pain relief. The woman takes deep breaths using a mouthpiece at the start of a contraction, then stops using it as the contraction eases. It can cause lightheadedness, nausea and sleepiness.

Intramuscular Pethidine or Diamorphine

Pethidine and diamorphine are **opioid** medications, usually given by **intramuscular injection**. They may help with anxiety and distress. They may cause drowsiness or nausea in the mother, and can cause respiratory depression in the neonate if given too close to birth. The effect on the baby may make the first feed more difficult.

Patient-Controlled Analgesia

Patients may be offered the option of patient-controlled intravenous **remifentanil**. This involves the patient pressing a button at the start of a contraction to administer a bolus of this short-acting opiate medication.

Patient-controlled analgesia requires careful monitoring. There needs to be input from an anaesthetist, and facilities in place if adverse events occur. This includes access to naloxone for respiratory depression, and atropine for bradycardia.

Epidural

An epidural involves inserting a small tube (catheter) into the **epidural space** in the lower back. This is **outside** the **dura mater**, separate from the **spinal cord** and **CSF**. **Local anaesthetic** medications are infused through the catheter into the **epidural space**, where they diffuse to the surrounding tissues, and through to the spinal cord where they have an analgesic effect. This offers good pain relief during labour. Anaesthetic options are **levobupivacaine** or **bupivacaine**, usually mixed with **fentanyl**.

Adverse effects:
- Headache after insertion
- Hypotension
- Motor weakness in the legs
- Nerve damage
- Prolonged second stage
- **Increased probability of instrumental delivery**

Women need urgent anaesthetic review if they develop significant **motor weakness** (unable to straight leg raise). The catheter may be incorrectly sited in the **subarachnoid space** (within the spinal cord), rather than the epidural space.

Umbilical Cord Prolapse

Cord prolapse is when the **umbilical cord** descends below the presenting part of the fetus and through the cervix into the vagina, after rupture of the fetal membranes. There is a significant danger of the presenting part compressing the cord, resulting in **fetal hypoxia**.

The most significant risk factor for cord prolapse is when the fetus is in an **abnormal lie** after 37 weeks gestation (i.e. unstable, transverse or oblique). Being in an abnormal lie provides space for the cord to prolapse below the presenting part. In a cephalic lie, the head typically descends into the pelvis, leaving no room for the cord to descend.

Diagnosis

Umbilical cord prolapse should be suspected where there are signs of fetal distress on the CTG. A prolapsed umbilical cord can be diagnosed by vaginal examination. Speculum examination can be used to confirm the diagnosis.

Management

Emergency caesarean section is indicated where cord prolapse occurs. A normal vaginal delivery has a high risk of cord compression and significant hypoxia to the baby. Pushing the cord back in is not recommended. The cord should be kept warm and wet and have minimal handling whilst waiting for delivery (handling causes vasospasm).

When the baby is compressing a prolapsed cord, the presenting part can be pushed upwards to prevent it compressing the cord. The woman can lie in the **left lateral position** (with a pillow under the hip) or the **knee-chest position** (on all fours), using gravity to draw the fetus away from the pelvis and reduce compression on the cord. **Tocolytic** medication (e.g. **terbutaline**) can be used to minimise contractions whilst waiting for delivery by caesarean section.

Shoulder Dystocia

Shoulder dystocia is when the **anterior shoulder** of the baby becomes stuck behind the **pubic symphysis** of the pelvis, after the head has been delivered. This requires additional obstetric manoeuvres to enable delivery of the rest of the body. Shoulder dystocia is an **obstetric emergency**.

Shoulder dystocia is often caused by **macrosomia** secondary to **gestational diabetes**.

Presentation

Shoulder dystocia presents with difficulty delivering the face and head, and obstruction in delivering the shoulders after delivery of the head. There may be **failure of restitution**, where the head remains face downwards (occipito-anterior) and does not turn sideways as expected after delivery of the head. The **turtle-neck sign** is where the head is delivered but then retracts back into the vagina.

Management

Shoulder dystocia is an obstetric emergency and needs to be managed by experienced midwives and obstetricians. The first step is to get help, including anaesthetics and paediatrics. Several techniques can be used to manage the condition and deliver the baby.

Episiotomy can be used to enlarge the vaginal opening and reduce the risk of perineal tears. It is not always necessary.

McRoberts manoeuvre involves hyperflexion of the mother at the hip (bringing her knees to her abdomen). This provides a **posterior pelvic tilt**, lifting the pubic symphysis up and out of the way.

Pressure to the anterior shoulder involves pressing on the suprapubic region of the abdomen. This puts pressure on the posterior aspect of the baby's anterior shoulder, to encourage it down and under the pubic symphysis.

Rubins manoeuvre involves reaching into the vagina to put pressure on the posterior aspect of the baby's anterior shoulder to help it move under the pubic symphysis.

Wood's screw manoeuvre is performed during a Rubins manoeuvre. The other hand is used to reach in the vagina and put pressure on the anterior aspect of the posterior shoulder. The top shoulder is pushed forwards, and the bottom shoulder is pushed backwards, rotating the baby and helping delivery. If this does not work, the reverse motion can be tried, pushing the top shoulder backwards and the bottom shoulder forwards.

Zavanelli manoeuver involves pushing the baby's head back into the vagina so that the baby can be delivered by emergency caesarean section.

Complications

The key complications of shoulder dystocia are:
- Fetal hypoxia (and subsequent cerebral palsy)
- Brachial plexus injury and Erb's palsy
- Perineal tears
- Postpartum haemorrhage

Instrumental Delivery

Instrumental delivery refers to a vaginal delivery assisted by either a **ventouse suction cup** or **forceps**. Tools are used to help deliver the baby's head. About 10% of births in the UK are assisted by an instrumental delivery.

The procedure can usually be carried out on the labour ward. However, if there are concerns about whether it will be successful, the woman may be moved to theatre so that rapid delivery by caesarean section can be performed if necessary.

A single dose of **co-amoxiclav** is recommended after instrumental delivery to reduce the risk of maternal infection.

Indications

The decision to perform an instrumental delivery is based on the clinical judgement of the midwife or obstetrician. Some key indications are:
- Failure to progress
- Fetal distress
- Maternal exhaustion
- Control of the head in various fetal positions

TOM TIP: It is worth remembering there is an increased risk of requiring an instrumental delivery when an epidural is in place for analgesia.

Risks

Having an instrumental delivery increases the risk to the mother of:
- Postpartum haemorrhage
- Episiotomy
- Perineal tears
- Injury to the anal sphincter
- Incontinence of the bladder or bowel
- Nerve injury (**obturator** or **femoral** nerve)

The key risks to remember to the baby are:
- **Cephalohaematoma** with **ventouse**
- **Facial nerve palsy** with **forceps**

Rarely there can be serious risks to the baby:
- Subgaleal haemorrhage (most dangerous)
- Intracranial haemorrhage
- Skull fracture
- Spinal cord injury

Ventouse

A ventouse is essentially a suction cup on a cord. The suction cup goes on the baby's head, and the doctor or midwife applies careful traction to the cord to help pull the baby out of the vagina.

The main complication for the baby is **cephalohaematoma**. This involves a collection of blood between the skull and the periosteum.

Forceps

Forceps look like large metal salad tongs. They come as two pieces of curved metal that attach together, go either side of the baby's head and grip the head in a way that allows the doctor or midwife to apply careful traction and pull the head from the vagina.

The main complication for the baby is **facial nerve palsy**, with **facial paralysis** on one side.

Forceps delivery can leave **bruises** on the baby's face. Rarely the baby can develop **fat necrosis**, leading to hardened lumps of fat on their cheeks. Fat necrosis resolves spontaneously over time.

Nerve Injuries

Rarely an instrumental delivery may result in **nerve injury** in the mother. This usually resolves over 6 - 8 weeks. The affected nerves may be:
- *Femoral nerve*
- *Obturator nerve*

The **femoral nerve** may be compressed against the inguinal canal during a forceps delivery. Injury to this nerve causes **weakness of knee extension**, loss of the **patella reflex** and **numbness** of the anterior thigh and medial lower leg.

The **obturator nerve** may be compressed by forceps during instrumental delivery or by the fetal head during normal delivery. Injury causes weakness of **hip adduction** and **rotation**, and **numbness** of the medial thigh.

Three other nerve injuries can occur during birth that are usually unrelated to instrumental delivery:
- *Lateral cutaneous nerve of the thigh*
- *Lumbosacral plexus*
- *Common peroneal nerve*

The **lateral cutaneous nerve of the thigh** runs under the **inguinal ligament**. Prolonged flexion at the hip while in the lithotomy position can result in injury, causing numbness of the anterolateral thigh.

The **lumbosacral plexus** may be compressed by the fetal head during the second stage of labour. Injury to this network of nerves nerve can cause **foot drop** and **numbness** of the anterolateral thigh, lower leg and foot.

The **common peroneal nerve** may be injured by compression on the head of the fibula whilst in the lithotomy position. Injury to this nerve causes **foot drop** and numbness in the lateral lower leg.

Perineal Tears

A perineal tear occurs where the external vaginal opening is too narrow to accommodate the baby. This leads to the skin and tissue in that area tearing as the baby's head passes.

Perineal tears can range from a graze, to a large tear involving the **anal sphincter** (third-degree) and **rectal mucosa** (fourth-degree).

Perineal tears are more common with:
- First births (nulliparity)
- Large babies (over 4kg)
- Shoulder dystocia
- Asian ethnicity
- Occipito-posterior position
- Instrumental deliveries

Classification

There are four degrees of perineal tear, each involving injury to tissue beyond the previous:
- **First-degree** - injury limited to the **frenulum of the labia minora** (where they meet posteriorly) and superficial skin
- **Second-degree** - including the **perineal muscles**, but not affecting the anal sphincter
- **Third-degree** - including the **anal sphincter**, but not affecting the rectal mucosa
- **Fourth-degree** - including the **rectal mucosa**

Third-degree tears can be subcategorised as:
- **3A** - less than 50% of the **external anal sphincter** affected
- **3B** - more than 50% of the **external anal sphincter** affected
- **3C** - external and internal anal sphincter affected

Management

First-degree tears usually do not require any sutures. When a perineal tear larger than first degree occurs, the mother usually requires sutures to correct the injury. A third or fourth-degree tear is likely to need repairing in theatre.

Additional measures are taken to reduce the risk of complications:
- **Broad-spectrum antibiotics** to reduce the risk of infection
- **Laxatives** to reduce the risk of constipation and wound dehiscence
- **Physiotherapy** to reduce the risk and severity of incontinence
- **Followup** to monitor for longstanding complications

Women that are symptomatic after third or fourth-degree tears are offered an **elective caesarean section** in subsequent pregnancies.

Complications

Short-term complications after repair include:
- Pain
- Infection
- Bleeding
- Wound dehiscence or wound breakdown

Perineal tears can lead to several lasting complications:
- Urinary incontinence
- Anal incontinence and altered bowel habit (third and fourth-degree tears)
- Fistula between the vagina and bowel (rare)
- Sexual dysfunction and dyspareunia (painful sex)
- Psychological and mental health consequences

Episiotomy

An episiotomy is where the obstetrician or midwife cuts the perineum before the baby is delivered. This is done in anticipation of needing additional room for delivery of the baby (e.g. before forceps delivery). It is performed under local anaesthetic. A cut is made at around 45 degrees diagonally, from the opening of the vagina downwards and laterally, to avoid damaging the anal sphincter. This is called a **mediolateral episiotomy**. The cut is sutured after delivery.

Perineal Massage

Perineal massage is a method for reducing the risk of perineal tears. It involves massaging the skin and tissues between the vagina and anus (perineum). This is done in a structured way from 34 weeks onwards to stretch and prepare the tissues for delivery.

Active Management of the Third Stage

The third stage of labour is from the completed birth of the baby to the delivery of the placenta. There are two options for the third stage:
- **Physiological management**
- **Active management**

Physiological management is where the placenta is delivered by maternal effort without medications or cord traction.

Active management of the third stage is where the midwife or doctor assist in delivering the placenta. It involves a dose of **intramuscular oxytocin** to help the uterus contract, and careful **traction** to the **umbilical cord** to guide the placenta out of the uterus and vagina. Active management shortens the third stage and reduces the risk of bleeding, but can be associated with **nausea and vomiting**.

Active management is routinely offered to all women to reduce the risk of postpartum haemorrhage. It is also initiated if there is:
- Haemorrhage
- More than a 60-minute delay in delivery of the placenta (prolonged third stage)

Steps

Active management of the third stage involves an **intramuscular** dose of **oxytocin** (10 IU) after delivery of the baby.

The cord is clamped and cut within 5 minutes of birth. There should be a delay of 1 - 3 minutes between delivery of the baby and clamping of the cord to allow blood to flow to the baby (unless the baby needs resuscitation).

The abdomen is palpated to assess for a uterine contraction before delivery of the placenta. **Controlled cord traction** is carefully applied during uterine contractions to help deliver the placenta, stopping if there is resistance. At the same time the other hand presses the uterus upwards (in the opposite direction) to prevent uterine prolapse. The aim is to deliver the placenta in one piece.

After delivery the uterus is massaged until it is contracted and firm. The placenta is examined to ensure it is complete and no tissue remains in the uterus.

Postpartum Haemorrhage

Postpartum haemorrhage (**PPH**) refers to bleeding after delivery of the baby and placenta. It is the most common cause of significant **obstetric haemorrhage**, and a potential cause of maternal death. To be classified as postpartum haemorrhage, there needs to be a loss of:
- 500ml after a vaginal delivery
- 1000ml after a caesarean section

It can be defined as:
- **Minor PPH** - under 1000ml blood loss
- **Major PPH** - over 1000ml blood loss
- **Moderate PPH** - 1000 - 2000ml blood loss
- **Severe PPH** - over 2000ml blood loss

It can also be categorised as:
- **Primary PPH** - bleeding within 24 hours of birth
- **Secondary PPH** - from 24 hours to 12 weeks after birth

Causes

There are four causes of postpartum haemorrhage, remembered using the "**Four Ts**" mnemonic:
- **Tone** (**uterine atony** - the most common cause)
- **Trauma** (e.g. perineal tear)
- **Tissue** (retained placenta)
- **Thrombin** (bleeding disorder)

Risk Factors

- Previous PPH
- Multiple pregnancy
- Obesity
- Large baby
- Failure to progress in the second stage of labour
- Prolonged third stage
- Pre-eclampsia
- Placenta accreta
- Retained placenta
- Instrumental delivery
- General anaesthesia
- Episiotomy or perineal tear

Preventative Measures

Several measures can reduce the risk and consequences of postpartum haemorrhage:
- **Treating anaemia** during the antenatal period
- Giving birth with an **empty bladder** (a full bladder reduces uterine contraction)
- **Active management of the third stage** (with **intramuscular oxytocin** in the third stage)
- **Intravenous tranexamic acid** can be used during caesarean section (in the third stage) in higher-risk patients

Management

Postpartum haemorrhage is an obstetric emergency and needs to be managed by an experienced team, involving senior midwives, obstetricians, anaesthetists, haematologists, blood bank staff and porters.

Labour and Delivery

Management to stabilise the patient involves:
- Resuscitation with an ABCDE approach
- Lie the woman flat, keep her warm and communicate with her and her partner
- Insert two large-bore cannulas
- Bloods for FBC, U&E and clotting screen
- Group and cross match 4 units
- Warmed IV fluid and blood resuscitation as required
- Oxygen (regardless of saturations)
- Fresh frozen plasma is used where there are clotting abnormalities or after 4 units of blood transfusion

In severe cases, activate the **major haemorrhage protocol**. Each hospital will have a major haemorrhage protocol, which gives rapid access to 4 units of crossmatched or O negative blood.

Treatment to Stop the Bleeding

The treatment options for stopping the bleeding can be categorised as:
- Mechanical
- Medical
- Surgical

Mechanical treatment options involve:
- **Rubbing the uterus** through the abdomen to stimulates a uterine contraction (referred to as "rubbing up the fundus")
- **Catheterisation** (bladder distention prevents uterus contractions)

Medical treatment options involve:
- **Oxytocin** (slow injection followed by continuous infusion)
- **Ergometrine** (intravenous or intramuscular) stimulates smooth muscle contraction (contraindicated in hypertension)
- **Carboprost** (intramuscular) is a **prostaglandin analogue** that stimulates uterine contraction (caution in asthma)
- **Misoprostol** (sublingual) is also a **prostaglandin analogue** that stimulates uterine contraction
- **Tranexamic acid** (intravenous) is an **antifibrinolytic** that reduces bleeding

TOM TIP: The intravenous infusion of oxytocin is given as 40 units in 500 mls. You may hear midwives or obstetricians referring only to "40 units" without specifying the drug. They are referring to an oxytocin infusion for PPH.

Medical treatment options involve:
- **Intrauterine balloon tamponade** - inserting an inflatable balloon into the uterus to press against the bleeding
- **B-Lynch suture** - putting a suture around the uterus to compress it
- **Uterine artery ligation** - ligation of one or more of the arteries supplying the uterus to reduce the blood flow
- **Hysterectomy** is the "last resort", but will stop the bleeding and may save the woman's life

Secondary Postpartum Haemorrhage

Secondary postpartum haemorrhage is where bleeding occurs from 24 hours to 12 weeks postpartum. This is more likely to be due to **retained products of conception** (**RPOC**) or **infection** (i.e. **endometritis**).

Investigations include:
- **Ultrasound** for retained products of conception
- **Endocervical** and **high vaginal swabs** for infection

Management depends on the cause:
- **Evacuation** of retained products of conception
- **Antibiotics** for infection

Caesarean Section

A caesarean section involves a surgical operation to deliver the baby via an incision in the abdomen and uterus. It can be a planned procedure (**elective caesarean**) or performed where there are acute problems during the antenatal period or labour (**emergency caesarean**).

Elective Caesarean

Elective caesarean section involves a planned date on which a woman will come in for delivery. It is usually performed under a **spinal anaesthetic**, and is considered generally a very safe and routine procedure. Usually these are performed after 39 weeks gestation.

Indications for elective caesarean include:
- Previous caesarean
- Symptomatic after a previous significant perineal tear
- Placenta praevia
- Vasa praevia
- Breech presentation
- Multiple pregnancy
- Uncontrolled HIV infection
- Cervical cancer

Emergency Caesarean

There are four categories of emergency caesarean section:
- **Category 1**: There is an immediate threat to the life of the mother or baby. Decision to delivery time is 30 minutes.
- **Category 2**: There is not an imminent threat to life, but caesarean is required urgently due to compromise of the mother or baby. Decision to delivery time is 75 minutes.
- **Category 3**: Delivery is required, but mother and baby are stable.
- **Category 4**: This is an elective caesarean, as described above.

Procedure

The most commonly used skin incision is a transverse lower uterine segment incision. There are two possible incisions:
- **Pfannenstiel incision** is a curved incision two fingers width above the pubic symphysis
- **Joel-Cohen incision** is a straight incision that is slightly higher (this is the recommended incision)

A **vertical incision** down the middle of the abdomen is also possible, but this is rarely used. It may be used in certain circumstances, such as very premature deliveries and anterior placenta praevia.

Blunt dissection is used after the initial incision with a scalpel, to separate the remaining layers of the abdominal wall and uterus. Blunt dissection involves using fingers, blunt instruments and traction to tear the tissues apart, rather than to cut them with sharp tools such as a scalpel. This results in less bleeding, shorter operating times and less risk of injury to the baby.

The layers of the abdomen that need to be dissected during a caesarean are:
- **Skin**
- **Subcutaneous tissue**
- **Fascia / rectus sheath** (the aponeurosis of the transversus abdominis and external and internal oblique muscles)
- **Rectus abdominis muscles** (separated vertically)
- **Peritoneum**
- **Vesicouterine peritoneum** (and bladder) - the bladder is separated from the uterus with a bladder flap
- **Uterus** (perimetrium, myometrium and endometrium)
- **Amniotic sac**

The baby is delivered by hand with the assistance of pressure on the fundus. Forceps may be used if necessary.

The uterus is closed inside the abdomen using **two layers** of sutures. **Exteriorisation** (taking the uterus out of the abdomen) is avoided if possible. The abdomen and skin are then closed.

Anaesthetic

A **spinal anaesthetic** involves giving an injection of a local anaesthetic (such as lidocaine) into the **cerebrospinal fluid** at the lower back. This blocks the nerves from the abdomen downwards.

A spinal anaesthetic is safer, and leads to fewer complications and a faster recovery than a general anaesthetic. The potential problems are that the patient remains awake (most patients tolerate this well, but some prefer to be asleep), and it takes longer to initiate than a general anaesthetic.

Risks associated with having an anaesthetic:
- Allergic reactions or anaphylaxis
- Hypotension
- Headache
- Urinary retention
- Nerve damage (spinal anaesthetic)
- Haematoma (spinal anaesthetic)
- Sore throat (general anaesthetic)
- Damage to the teeth or mouth (general anaesthetic)

Complications

Elective caesarean sections are generally considered a very safe and routine procedure. Emergency caesarean sections have a higher risk of complications, as they are usually performed in less controlled settings and for more acute indications (e.g. fetal distress). There are a long list of potential complications, as with any surgery.

Measures to reduce the risks during caesarean section are:
- **H2 receptor antagonists** (e.g. ranitidine) or **proton pump inhibitors** (e.g. omeprazole) before the procedure
- **Prophylactic antibiotics** during the procedure to reduce the risk of infection
- **Oxytocin** during the procedure to reduce the risk of postpartum haemorrhage
- **Venous thromboembolism** (VTE) prophylaxis with low molecular weight heparin

There is a risk of aspiration pneumonitis during caesarean section, caused by acid reflux and aspiration during the prolonged period lying flat. **H2 receptor antagonists** (e.g. **ranitidine**) or **proton pump inhibitors** (e.g. **omeprazole**) are given before the procedure to reduce the risk of this happening.

Generic surgical risks:
- Bleeding
- Infection
- Pain
- Venous thromboembolism

Complications in the postpartum period:
- Postpartum haemorrhage
- Wound infection
- Wound dehiscence
- Endometritis

Damage to local structures:
- Ureter
- Bladder
- Bowel
- Blood vessels

Effects on the abdominal organs:
- Ileus
- Adhesions
- Hernias

Effects on future pregnancies:
- Increased risk of repeat caesarean
- Increased risk of uterine rupture
- Increased risk of placenta praevia
- Increased risk of stillbirth

Effects on the baby:
- Risk of lacerations (about 2%)
- Increased incidence of transient tachypnoea of the newborn

Vaginal Birth After Caesarean (VBAC)

It is possible to have a vaginal birth after a previous caesarean section, provided the cause of the caesarean is unlikely to recur. An assessment of the likelihood of success should be made in each case. Success rate of VBAC is around 75%. Uterine rupture risk in VBAC is about 0.5%.

Contraindications:
- Previous uterine rupture
- Classical caesarean scar (a vertical incision)
- Other usual contraindications to vaginal delivery (e.g. placenta praevia)

Venous Thromboembolism

Having a caesarean section is likely to lead to a period of reduced mobility. Women should have a VTE risk assessment performed to determine the type and duration of VTE prophylaxis (follow local guidelines). Prophylaxis for VTE involves:
- Early mobilisation
- Anti-embolism stockings or intermittent pneumatic compression of the legs
- Low molecular weight heparin (e.g. enoxaparin)

Maternal Sepsis

Sepsis is a condition where the body launches a large immune response to an infection, causing **systemic inflammation** and affecting organ function. It is a significant cause of maternal death.

Severe sepsis is when sepsis results in organ dysfunction, such as **hypoxia**, **oliguria** or **raised lactate**. **Septic shock** is defined when arterial blood pressure drops, causing organ hypo-perfusion.

Sepsis in pregnancy is a medical emergency that requires prompt recognition and management to reduce the risk of maternal and fetal morbidity and mortality.

Two key causes of sepsis in pregnancy are:
- **Chorioamnionitis**
- **Urinary tract infections**

Chorioamnionitis

Chorioamnionitis is an infection of the **chorioamniotic membranes** and **amniotic fluid**. Chorioamnionitis is a leading cause of maternal sepsis and a notable cause of maternal death (along with urinary tract infection). It usually occurs in later pregnancy and during labour.

Chorioamnionitis can be caused by a large variety of bacteria, including **gram-positive bacteria**, **gram-negative bacteria** and **anaerobes**.

Presentation

All patients admitted to maternity inpatient units, such as at the antenatal ward and labour ward, will have monitoring on a **MEOWS chart**. MEOWS stands for **maternity early obstetric warning system**. This includes monitoring their physical observations to identify signs of sepsis.

The non-specific signs of **sepsis** include:
- Fever
- Tachycardia
- Raised respiratory rate (often an early sign)
- Reduced oxygen saturations
- Low blood pressure
- Altered consciousness
- Reduced urine output
- Raised white blood cells on a full blood count
- Evidence of fetal compromise on a CTG

Additional signs and symptoms related to **chorioamnionitis** include:
- Abdominal pain
- Uterine tenderness
- Vaginal discharge

Additional signs and symptoms related to a **urinary tract infection** include:
- Dysuria
- Urinary frequency
- Suprapubic pain or discomfort
- Renal angle pain (with pyelonephritis)
- Vomiting (with pyelonephritis)

Investigations

Arrange blood tests for patients with suspected sepsis:
- **Full blood count** to assess cell count including white cells and neutrophils
- **U&Es** to assess kidney function and for acute kidney injury
- **LFTs** to assess liver function and as a possible source of infection (e.g. acute cholecystitis)
- **CRP** to assess inflammation
- **Clotting** to assess for disseminated intravascular coagulopathy (DIC)
- **Blood cultures** to assess for bacteraemia
- **Blood gas** to assess **lactate**, pH and glucose

Additional investigations can be helpful based on the suspected source of infection:
- Urine dipstick and culture
- High vaginal swab
- Throat swab
- Sputum culture
- Wound swab
- Lumbar puncture for meningitis or encephalitis

Management

Senior obstetricians and midwives should be involved early in the care of women with suspected chorioamnionitis or sepsis. There should be a local guideline in your hospital for the management of maternal sepsis. Early recognition and management is essential. This will involve the **septic six** (see below).

Continuous **maternal** and **fetal monitoring** is required. Depending on the condition of the mother and fetus, early delivery may be needed. Emergency caesarean section may be indicated when there is fetal distress, guided by a senior obstetrician. **General anaesthesia** is usually required for women with sepsis, as spinal anaesthesia is avoided.

Always follow the local guidelines when choosing antibiotics. Very heavy-hitting antibiotics are required, needing to cover gram-positive, gram-negative and anaerobes. There are also significant consequences of inadequate treatment. Example regimes include **piperacillin and tazobactam** (**tazocin**) plus **gentamicin**, or **amoxicillin**, **clindamycin** and **gentamicin**.

TOM TIP: When preparing for exams and thinking about possible antibiotic choices for different conditions, it is worth searching google for local NHS trust antibiotic policies. It is interesting to see how they vary between trusts, given the differences in antibiotic resistance in different locations. Think about what specific bacteria the microbiologists are targeting with varying choices of antibiotics.

Septic Six

Three tests:
- Blood lactate level
- Blood cultures
- Urine output

Three treatments:
- Oxygen to maintain oxygen saturations 94-98%
- Empirical broad-spectrum antibiotics
- IV fluids

Amniotic Fluid Embolisation

Amniotic fluid embolisation is a rare (2 per 100,000 deliveries) but severe condition where the amniotic fluid passes into the mother's blood. This usually occurs around labour and delivery. The amniotic fluid contains fetal tissue, causing an immune reaction from the mother. This immune reaction to cells from the fetus leads to a systemic illness. It has more similarities to anaphylaxis than venous thromboembolism. The mortality rate is around 20% or above.

Risk Factors

The main risk factors for amniotic fluid embolus are:
- Increasing maternal age
- Induction of labour
- Caesarean section
- Multiple pregnancy

Presentation

Amniotic fluid embolisation usually presents around the time of labour and delivery, but can be postpartum. It can present similarly to sepsis, pulmonary embolism or anaphylaxis, with an acute onset of symptoms of:
- Shortness of breath
- Hypoxia
- Hypotension
- Coagulopathy
- Haemorrhage
- Tachycardia
- Confusion
- Seizures
- Cardiac arrest

Management

The overall management of amniotic fluid embolism is **supportive**. There are no specific treatments.

Amniotic fluid embolism is a medical emergency. It requires the input of experienced obstetricians, physicians, anaesthetists, intensive care teams and haematologists. They are likely to need transfer to the ***intensive care unit***.

The initial management of any acutely unwell patient is with an ABCDE approach, assessing and treating:
- ***A – Airway***: Secure the airway
- ***B – Breathing***: Provide oxygen for hypoxia
- ***C – Circulation***: IV fluids to treat hypotension and blood transfusion in haemorrhage
- ***D – Disability***: Treat seizures and consider other neurological deficits
- ***E – Exposure***

Cardiopulmonary resuscitation and immediate caesarean section are required if cardiac arrest occurs.

Uterine Rupture

Uterine rupture is a complication of labour, where the muscle layer of the uterus (myometrium) ruptures. With an *incomplete rupture* (*uterine dehiscence*), the *uterine serosa* (*perimetrium*) surrounding the uterus remains intact. With a *complete rupture*, the serosa ruptures along with the myometrium, and the contents of the uterus are released into the *peritoneal cavity*.

Uterine rupture leads to significant bleeding. The baby may be released from the uterus into the peritoneal cavity. It has a high morbidity and mortality for both the baby and mother.

Risk factors

The main *risk factor* for uterine rupture is a *previous caesarean section*. The scar on the uterus becomes a point of weakness, and may rupture with excessive pressure (e.g. excessive stimulation by oxytocin). It is extremely rare for uterine rupture to occur in a patient that is giving birth for the first time.

The risk factors to consider are:
- Vaginal birth after caesarean (VBAC)
- Previous uterine surgery
- Increased BMI
- High parity
- Increased age
- Induction of labour
- Use of oxytocin to stimulate contractions

Presentation

Uterine rupture presents with an acutely unwell mother and *abnormal CTG*. It may occur with induction or augmentation of labour, with signs and symptoms of:
- Abdominal pain
- Vaginal bleeding
- **Ceasing of uterine contractions**
- Hypotension
- Tachycardia
- Collapse

Management

Uterine rupture is an obstetric emergency. Resuscitation and transfusion may be required. *Emergency caesarean section* is necessary to remove the baby, stop any bleeding and repair or remove the uterus (hysterectomy).

Uterine Inversion

Uterine inversion is a rare complication of birth, where the **fundus of the uterus** drops down through the uterine cavity and cervix, turning the uterus inside out. It is a very rare occurrence, and you are unlikely to see one in your career unless you become a midwife or obstetrician. It is a life-threatening obstetric emergency.

Incomplete uterine inversion (partial inversion) is where the fundus descends inside the uterus or vagina, but not as far as the *introitus* (opening of the vagina). *Complete uterine inversion* involves the uterus descending through the vagina to the introitus.

Uterine inversion may be the result of pulling too hard on the umbilical cord during active management of the third stage of labour.

Presentation

Uterine inversion typically presents with a large **postpartum haemorrhage**. There may be **maternal shock** or **collapse**.

An incomplete uterine inversion may be felt with manual vaginal examination. With a complete uterine inversion, the uterus may be seen at the introitus of the vagina.

Management

There are three options for treating uterine inversion:
- Johnson manoeuvre
- Hydrostatic methods
- Surgery

Initial management of an inverted uterus is with the **Johnson manoeuvre**, which involves using a hand to push the fundus back up into the abdomen and the correct position. The whole hand and most of the forearm will be inserted into the vagina to return the fundus to the correct position. It is held in place for several minutes, and medications are used to create a uterine contraction (i.e. oxytocin). The ligaments and uterus need to generate enough tension to remain in place.

Where the Johnson manoeuvre fails, **hydrostatic methods** can be used. This involves filling the vagina with fluid to "inflate" the uterus back to the normal position. It requires a tight seal at the entrance of the vagina, which can be challenging to achieve.

Where both non-surgical methods fail, **surgery** is required. A laparotomy is performed (opening the abdomen) and the uterus is returned to the normal position.

Other measures to stabilise the mother and treat the consequences may be required. For example, they may require resuscitation, treatment of postpartum haemorrhage and blood transfusion.

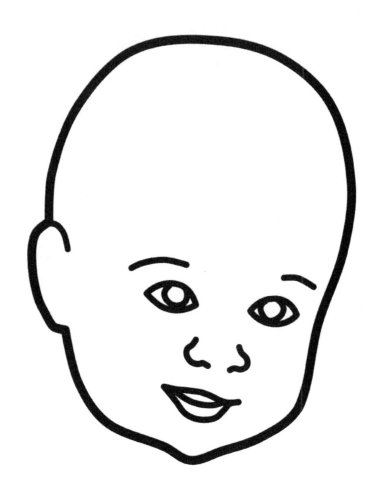

POSTNATAL CARE

10.1	Routine Postnatal Care	223
10.2	Postpartum Endometritis	224
10.3	Retained Products of Conception	225
10.4	Postpartum Anaemia	226
10.5	Postnatal Depression	227
10.6	Lactational Mastitis	228
10.7	Postpartum Thyroiditis	229
10.8	Sheehan's Syndrome	231

Routine Postnatal Care

Most women will have routine midwife-led care in the postnatal period. They may be transferred to the postnatal ward for a short period of monitoring and adjustment after delivery.

In the days after delivery they will have:
- Analgesia as required
- Help establishing breast or bottle-feeding
- Venous thromboembolism risk assessment
- Monitoring for postpartum haemorrhage
- Monitoring for sepsis
- Monitoring blood pressure (after pre-eclampsia)
- Monitoring recovery after a caesarean or perineal tear
- Full blood count check (after bleeding, caesarean or antenatal anaemia)
- Anti-D for rhesus D negative women (depending on the baby's blood group)
- Routine baby check

After the initial postnatal period, they will have routine follow up with a midwife to discuss topics such as:
- General wellbeing
- Mood and depression
- Bleeding and menstruation
- Urinary incontinence and pelvic floor exercises
- Scar healing after episiotomy or caesarean
- Contraception
- Breastfeeding
- Vaccines (e.g. MMR)

Six-Week Postnatal Check

A routine six-week postnatal appointment is commonly offered by GP practices to check how the mother is doing. It is usually done at the same time as the six-week newborn baby check.

The topics that are covered at the six-week check include:
- General wellbeing
- Mood and depression
- Bleeding and menstruation
- Scar healing after episiotomy or caesarean
- Contraception
- Breastfeeding
- Fasting blood glucose (after gestational diabetes)
- Blood pressure (after hypertension or pre-eclampsia)
- Urine dipstick for protein (after pre-eclampsia)

Menstruation After Delivery

In the period shortly after birth, there will be vaginal bleeding as the endometrium initially breaks down, then returns to normal over time. This is a mix of blood, endometrial tissue and mucus, and is called **lochia**. Initially, it will be a dark red colour. Over time will turn brown and become lighter in flow and colour. Tampons should be avoided during this period, as they carry a risk of infection. Bleeding should settle within six weeks.

Breastfeeding releases oxytocin, which causes the uterus to contract, leading to slightly more bleeding during episodes of breastfeeding. This is normal.

Women who are breastfeeding may not have a return to regular menstrual periods for six months or longer (unless they stop breastfeeding). The absence of periods related to breastfeeding is called **lactational amenorrhoea**.

Bottle-feeding women will begin having menstrual periods from 3 weeks onwards. This is unpredictable, and periods can be delayed or irregular at first.

Contraception After Childbirth

Fertility is not considered to return until **21 days** after giving birth, and contraception is not required up to this point. The risk of pregnancy is very low before 21 days. After 21 days women are considered fertile, and will need contraception (including condoms for seven days when starting the combined pill or two days for progestogen-only contraception).

Lactational amenorrhea is over 98% effective as contraception for up to 6 months after birth. Women must be **fully breastfeeding** and **amenorrhoeic** (no periods).

The **progestogen-only pill** and **implant** are considered safe in breastfeeding and can be started at any time after birth.

The **combined contraceptive pill** should be avoided in breastfeeding (UKMEC 4 before six weeks postpartum, UKMEC 2 after six weeks).

A **copper coil** or **intrauterine system** (e.g. Mirena) can be inserted either within 48 hours of birth or more than four weeks after birth (UKMEC 1), but not inserted between 48 hours and four weeks of delivery (UKMEC 3).

TOM TIP: Remember that the combined pill should not be started before six weeks after childbirth in women that are breastfeeding. The progestogen-only pill or implant can be started any time after birth.

Postpartum Endometritis

Endometritis refers to **inflammation** of the **endometrium**, usually caused by **infection**. It can occur in the **postpartum period**, as infection is introduced during or after labour and delivery. The process of delivery opens the uterus and allows bacteria from the vagina to travel upwards and infect the endometrium.

Endometritis occurs more commonly after **caesarean section** compared with vaginal delivery. **Prophylactic antibiotics** are given during a caesarean to reduce the risk of infection.

Endometritis can be caused by a large variety of **gram-negative**, **gram-positive** and **anaerobic** bacteria. It can also be caused by **sexually transmitted infections** such as **chlamydia** and **gonorrhoea**.

When endometritis occurs unrelated to pregnancy and delivery, it is usually part of pelvic inflammatory disease, which is covered elsewhere.

Presentation

Postpartum endometritis can present from shortly after birth to several weeks postpartum. It presents with:
- Foul-smelling discharge or lochia
- Bleeding that gets heavier or does not improve with time
- Lower abdominal or pelvic pain
- Fever
- Sepsis

Diagnosis and Management

Investigations to help establish the diagnosis include:
- **Vaginal swabs** (including chlamydia and gonorrhoea if there are risk factors)
- **Urine culture** and **sensitivities**

Ultrasound may be considered to rule out **retained products of conception**. Ultrasound is not helping in diagnosing endometritis.

Septic patients will require hospital admission and the **septic six**, including blood cultures and broad-spectrum IV antibiotics (according to local guidelines). A combination of clindamycin and gentamicin is often recommended. Blood tests will show signs of infection (e.g. raised WBC and CRP).

Patients presenting with milder symptoms and no signs of sepsis may be treated in the community with oral antibiotics. A typical choice of broad-spectrum oral antibiotic might be co-amoxiclav, depending on the risk of chlamydia and gonorrhoea.

Retained Products of Conception

Retained products of conception refers to when pregnancy-related tissue (e.g. placental tissue or fetal membranes) remain in the uterus after delivery. It can also occur after miscarriage or termination of pregnancy.

Placenta accreta is a significant risk factor for retained products of conception.

Presentation

Retained products of conception may be present in patients without any suggestive symptoms. It can present with:
- **Vaginal bleeding** that gets heavier or does not improve with time
- Abnormal vaginal discharge
- Lower abdominal or pelvic pain
- **Fever** (if infection occurs)

Diagnosis

Ultrasound is the investigation of choice for confirming the diagnosis.

Management

The standard management of postpartum retained products of conception is to remove them surgically.

Evacuation of retained products of conception (**ERPC**) is a surgical procedure involving a **general anaesthetic**. The **cervix** is gradually widened using dilators, and the retained products are manually removed through the cervix using **vacuum aspiration** and **curettage** (scraping). The procedure may be referred to as "**dilatation and curettage**". Two key complications are:
- Endometritis
- Asherman's syndrome

Asherman's syndrome is where **adhesions** (sometimes called **synechiae**) form **within the uterus**. **Endometrial curettage** (scraping) can damage the **basal layer** of the **endometrium**. This damaged tissue can heal abnormally, creating scar tissue (adhesions) connecting areas of the uterus that are not normally connected. There may be adhesions binding the uterine walls together, or within the endocervix, sealing it shut. This can lead to amenorrhoea and infertility.

Postpartum Anaemia

Postpartum anaemia is defined as a **haemoglobin** of less than 100 g/l in the postpartum period. Anaemia is common after delivery due to acute blood loss.

Most women lose some blood during delivery. In complicated deliveries, caesarean sections and postpartum haemorrhage, women can lose upwards of 1.5 litres of blood. It is essential to optimise the treatment of anaemia during pregnancy, so that women have optimal haemoglobin and iron stores before delivery.

Management

A **full blood count** is checked the day after delivery if there has been:
- Postpartum haemorrhage over 500ml
- Caesarean section
- Antenatal anaemia
- Symptoms of anaemia

Treatment of anaemia is based on individual factors and preferences, alongside local guidelines. As a rough guide (local policies will vary):
- Hb under 100 g/l - start **oral iron** (e.g. ferrous sulphate 200mg three times daily for three months)
- Hb under 90 g/l - consider an **iron infusion** in addition to oral iron (e.g. **Monofer**, **CosmoFer** or **Ferinject**)
- Hb under 70 g/l - **blood transfusion** in addition to oral iron

An iron infusion is also considered in women that:
- May have poor adherence to oral treatment
- Cannot tolerate oral iron
- Fail to respond to oral iron
- Cannot absorb oral iron (e.g. inflammatory bowel disease)

Iron infusions carry a risk of allergic and anaphylactic reactions. They should be used with particular caution in patients with a history of allergy or asthma.

TOM TIP: It is worth noting that active infection is a contraindication to an iron infusion. Many pathogens "feed" on iron, meaning that intravenous iron can lead to proliferation of the pathogen and worsening infection. It is important to wait until the infection is treated before giving an iron infusion.

Postnatal Depression

Postnatal depression is characterised by low mood in the postnatal period.

There is a spectrum of postnatal mental health issues:
- **Baby blues** is seen in the majority of women in the **first week** or so after birth
- **Postnatal depression** is seen in about **one in ten** women, with a peak around **three months** after birth
- **Puerperal psychosis** is seen in about **one in a thousand** women, starting **a few weeks** after birth

Baby Blues

Baby blues affect more than 50% of women in the first week or so after birth, particularly first-time mothers. It presents with symptoms such as:
- Mood swings
- Low mood
- Anxiety
- Irritability
- Tearfulness

Baby blues may be the result of a combination of:
- Significant hormonal changes
- Recovery from birth
- Fatigue and sleep deprivation
- The responsibility of caring for the neonate
- Establishing feeding
- All the other changes and events around this time

Symptoms are usually mild, only last a few days and resolve within two weeks of delivery. No treatment is required.

Postnatal Depression

Postnatal depression is similar to depression that occurs outside of pregnancy, with the classic triad of:
- Low mood
- **Anhedonia** (lack of pleasure in activities)
- Low energy

Typically, women are affected around three months after birth. Symptoms should last at least two weeks before postnatal depression is diagnosed.

Treatment is similar to depression at other times:
- **Mild cases** may be managed with additional support, self-help and follow up with their GP
- **Moderate cases** may be managed with antidepressant medications (e.g. SSRIs) and cognitive behavioural therapy
- **Severe cases** may need input from specialist psychiatry services, and rarely inpatient care on the mother and baby unit

Edinburgh Postnatal Depression Scale

The Edinburgh postnatal depression scale can be used to assess how the mother has felt over the past week, as a screening tool for postnatal depression.

There are ten questions, with a total score out of 30 points. A score of 10 or more suggests postnatal depression.

Puerperal Psychosis

Puerperal psychosis is a rare but severe illness that typically has an onset between two to three weeks after delivery. Women experience full psychotic symptoms, such as:

- Delusions
- Hallucinations
- Depression
- Mania
- Confusion
- Thought disorder

Women with puerperal psychosis need urgent assessment and input from specialist mental health services.

Treatment is directed by specialist services, and may involve:
- Admission to the **mother and baby unit**
- Cognitive behavioural therapy
- Medications (**antidepressants**, **antipsychotics** or **mood stabilisers**)
- Electroconvulsive therapy (ECT)

Mother and Baby Unit

The mother and baby unit is a specialist unit for pregnant women and women that have given birth in the past 12 months. They are designed so that the mother and baby can remain together and continue to bond. Mothers are supported to continue caring for their baby while they get specialist treatment.

Preparation During Pregnancy

Women that have existing mental health concerns before or during pregnancy are referred to **perinatal mental health services** for advice and specialist input. This includes initiation and ongoing management of psychiatric medications, such as SSRIs, antipsychotics and lithium. A plan is put in place for after delivery to ensure they are followed up closely with help from midwives, health visitors, GPs, family and friends, so that treatment and additional support can be put in place early if required.

SSRI antidepressants taken during pregnancy can lead to **neonatal abstinence syndrome** (also known as **neonatal adaptation syndrome**). This presents in the first few days after birth with symptoms such as irritability and poor feeding. Neonates are monitored for this after delivery. Supportive management is usually all that is required.

Lactational Mastitis

Mastitis refers to **inflammation** of breast tissue, and is a common complication of **breastfeeding**. It can occur with or without associated infection.

Mastitis can be caused by **obstruction** in the ducts and accumulation of milk. Regularly expressing breast milk can help prevent this occurring.

Mastitis can also be caused by **infection**. Bacteria can enter at the nipple and back-track into the ducts, causing infection and inflammation. The most common bacteria is **staph aureus**.

Presentation

Mastitis presents with:
- Breast pain and tenderness (unilateral)
- Erythema in a focal area of breast tissue
- Local warmth and inflammation
- Nipple discharge
- Fever

Management

Where mastitis is caused by blockage of the ducts, management is conservative, with continued breastfeeding, expressing milk and breast massage. Heat packs, warm showers and simple analgesia can help symptoms.

When conservative management is not effective, or infection is suspected (e.g. they have a fever), antibiotics should be started. **Flucloxacillin** is first line, or erythromycin if allergic to penicillin. A sample of milk can be sent to the lab for **culture and sensitivities**. **Fluconazole** may be used for suspected **candidal** infections.

Women should be encouraged to continue breastfeeding, even when infection is suspected. It will not harm the baby and will help to clear the mastitis by encouraging flow. Where breastfeeding is difficult, or there is milk left after feeding, they can express milk to empty the breast.

A rare complication if not adequately treated, is a **breast abscess**. This may need surgical **incision and drainage**.

Candida of the Nipple

Candidal infection of the nipple can occur, often **after a course of antibiotics**. This can lead to **recurrent mastitis**, as it causes cracked skin on the nipple that creates an entrance for infection. It is associated with **oral thrush** and **candidal nappy rash** in the infant.

Candida infection of the nipple may present with:
- Sore nipples bilaterally, particularly after feeding
- Nipple tenderness and itching
- Cracked, flaky or shiny areola
- Symptoms in the baby, such as white patches in the mouth and on the tongue, or candidal nappy rash

Both the mother and baby need treatment, or it will reoccur. Treatment is with:
- **Topical miconazole** 2% to the nipple after each breastfeed
- Treatment for the baby (e.g. oral **miconazole gel** or **nystatin**)

Postpartum Thyroiditis

Postpartum thyroiditis is a condition where there are changes in thyroid function within 12 months of delivery, affecting women without a history of thyroid disease. It can involve **thyrotoxicosis** (hyperthyroidism), **hypothyroidism**, or both.

Over time the thyroid function returns to normal, and the patient will become asymptomatic again. A small portion of women will remain hypothyroid and need long-term thyroid hormone replacement.

Pathophysiology

The cause of postpartum thyroiditis is not clear. The leading theory is that pregnancy has an *immunosuppressant* effect on the mother's body that prevents her from rejecting the fetus. Once delivery has occurred, there can be an exaggerated rebound effect, with increased immune system activity and expression of antibodies. This may include antibodies that affect the thyroid gland, for example, *thyroid peroxidase antibodies*. These antibodies cause inflammation of the thyroid gland, leading to over or under-activity.

Stages

There is a typical pattern of postpartum thyroiditis. Not all women will follow this pattern. There are three stages:
1. **Thyrotoxicosis** (usually in the first three months)
2. **Hypothyroid** (usually from 3 - 6 months)
3. Thyroid function gradually **returns to normal** (usually within one year)

Signs and Symptoms

The signs and symptoms of thyrotoxicosis (hyperthyroidism) include:
- Anxiety and irritability
- Sweating and heat intolerance
- Tachycardia
- Weight loss
- Fatigue
- Frequent loose stools

The signs and symptoms of hypothyroidism include:
- Weight gain
- Fatigue
- Dry skin
- Coarse hair and hair loss
- Low mood
- Fluid retention (oedema, pleural effusions, ascites)
- Heavy or irregular periods
- Constipation

Thyroid Function Tests

In *thyrotoxicosis*, you expect **raised T3 and T4** and **suppressed TSH**. In *hypothyroidism*, you expect **low T3 and T4** and **raised TSH**.

Thyroid Status	TSH	T3 and T4
Hyperthyroidism	Low	High
Hypothyroidism	High	Low

Management

There should be a low threshold for testing thyroid function in women presenting with suggestive symptoms, particularly postnatal depression. Thyroid function tests are performed 6 - 8 weeks after delivery.

Patients with abnormal thyroid function tests in the postpartum period require referral to an endocrinologist for specialist management. Typical treatment is with:
- Thyrotoxicosis: **symptomatic control**, such as **propranolol** (a non-selective beta-blocker)
- Hypothyroidism: **levothyroxine**

Symptoms and thyroid function tests are monitored, and treatment is altered or stopped as the condition changes and improves.

Women with postpartum thyroiditis require **annual monitoring** of thyroid function tests, even after the condition has resolved. Monitoring is to identify those that go on to develop long-term hypothyroidism.

Sheehan's Syndrome

Sheehan's syndrome is a rare complication of **post-partum haemorrhage**, where the drop in circulating blood volume leads to **avascular necrosis** of the **pituitary gland**. Low blood pressure and reduced perfusion of the pituitary gland leads to **ischaemia** in the cells of the pituitary, and cell death.

Sheehan's syndrome only affects the **anterior pituitary gland**. Therefore, hormones produced by the posterior pituitary are spared.

Blood Supply

The anterior pituitary gets its blood supply from a low-pressure system called the **hypothalamo-hypophyseal portal system**. This system is susceptible to rapid drops in blood pressure.

The posterior pituitary gets a good blood supply from various arteries, and is therefore not susceptible to ischaemia when there is a drop in blood pressure.

Hormones

The *anterior pituitary* releases:
- **Thyroid-stimulating hormone (TSH)**
- **Adrenocorticotropic hormone (ACTH)**
- **Follicle-stimulating hormone (FSH)**
- **Luteinising hormone (LH)**
- **Growth hormone (GH)**
- **Prolactin**

The *posterior pituitary* releases (not affected in Sheehan's syndrome):
- **Oxytocin**
- **Antidiuretic hormone (ADH)**

Presentation

Sheehan's syndrome causes a lack of the hormones produced by the anterior pituitary, leading to signs and symptoms of:
- **Reduced lactation** (lack of prolactin)
- **Amenorrhea** (lack of LH and FSH)
- **Adrenal insufficiency** and **adrenal crisis**, caused by **low cortisol** (lack of ACTH)
- **Hypothyroidism** with **low thyroid hormones** (lack of TSH)

Management

Sheehan's syndrome will be managed under the guidance of a specialist endocrinologist. It will involve replacement for the missing hormones:
- **Oestrogen** and **progesterone** as hormone replacement therapy for the female sex hormones (until menopause)
- **Hydrocortisone** for adrenal insufficiency
- **Levothyroxine** for hypothyroidism
- **Growth hormone**

INDEX

Abortion 142
Acanthosis nigricans 47
Accelerations (CTG) 198
ACE inhibitors 154
Aciclovir 96
Actinomyces-like organisms 73, 119
Active management third stage 211
Acute fatty liver 178
Adenomyosis 36
Adhesions 34
Alcohol in pregnancy 149
Alkaline phosphatase 16
Amenorrhoea 21, 23
Amies transport medium 86
Amniocentesis 151
Amniotic fluid embolisation 219
Anaemia postpartum 226
Anaemia in pregnancy 166
Androgen insensitivity syndrome 69
Anovulation 126
Antenatal appointments 148
Antenatal steroids 195
Anti-D 158
Anticholinergic medications 62
Antral follicles 8
Aortocaval compression 189
Argyll-Robertson pupil 101
Aromatase 7
Artificial rupture of membranes 196
Asherman's syndrome 54
Atosiban 195, 200
Atrophic vaginitis 63
Avastin 75
B-Lynch suture 213
Baby blues 227
Bacterial vaginosis 83
Balloon tamponade 213
Balloon thermal ablation 30
Barrier methods 106
Bartholin's cyst 64
Beta-blockers 153
Bevacizumab 75
Bicornuate uterus 68
Bishop score 196
Black cohosh 41
Bladder diary 61
Blastocele 11
Blastocyst 11
Booking clinic 150
Braxton-Hicks contractions 18, 192
Breech 186
CA125 blood test 52
Caesarean section 214

Candida of the nipple 229
Candidiasis 84
Carboprost 202
Cardiac arrest 189
Cardinal movements of labour 19
Cardiotocography 197
Cerclage of the cervix 193
Cervical cancer 71
Cervical caps 106
Cervical cerclage 193
Cervical ectropion 55
Cervical intraepithelial neoplasia 72
Cervical ripening balloon 196
Cervical screening 72
Chancre 100
Changes in pregnancy 15
Chickenpox 156
Chlamydia 86
Chlamydial conjunctivitis 89
Chorioamnionitis 217
Chorion 12
Chorionic villi 13
Chorionic villus sampling 151
Clomifene 127
Clonidine 41
Co-cyprindiol 49
Coils 117
Colpitis maculassi 94
Colposcopy 73
Combined pill 107
Conception 10
Condoms 106
Condylomata lata 101
Cone biopsy 74
Congenital adrenal hyperplasia 24
Consent to contraception 122
Contraception 104
Copper coil 117, 120
Corpus luteum 10
Corpus luteum cyst 50
Cortisol 15
CT pulmonary angiogram 170
Culposuspension 62
Cyproterone 49
Cystocele 57
Cytomegalovirus 156
D-dimer 170
Decelerations (CTG) 198
Deep vein thrombosis 168
Delayed cord clamping 194
Dental dams 107
Depression 227
Dermoid cyst 51, 78

Diabetic retinopathy 175
Diamorphine 205
Diaphragms 106
Differential diagnosis 21
Dinoprostone 196
Dong quai 41
Down's syndrome 151
DVT 168
Dyskaryosis 72
Dysmenorrhoea 22
Ebstein's anomaly 155
Eclampsia 171
Ectopic pregnancy 135
Ectopy (cervix) 55
Eflornithine 49
Embryology 12
Embryonic disc 12
Embyroblast 11
Emergency contraception 120
Endometrial ablation 30
Endometrial cancer 48, 75
Endometrial hyperplasia 75
Endometrioma 51
Endometriosis 33
Endometritis 224
Entonox 205
Epidural 206
Epilepsy in pregnancy 152
Episiotomy 211
Ergometrine 201
Erosion (cervix) 55
ERPC 140
Evening primrose oil 41
Failure to progress 202
Female genital mutilation 66
Fertilisation 10
Fetal alcohol syndrome 149
Fetal fibronectin 194
Fetal growth restriction 159
Fetal pole 12
FGM 66
Fibroids 31
Fibronectin 194
Filshie clips 122
Finasteride 49
Fitz-Hugh-Curtis syndrome 93
Flutamide 49
Folic acid 149
Follicle-stimulating hormone 6, 15
Follicles 9
Follicular cyst 50
Follicular phase 8
Forceps 209

Frazer guidelines 123
FSH 6
Gardasil 75
Gardnerella vaginalis 83
Gas and air 205
Genital herpes 95
Germ cell tumours 51, 78
Gestational diabetes 174
Gillick competence 123
Ginseng 41
GnRH 6
Gonadotropin-releasing hormone 6
Gonococcal conjunctivitis 91
Gonorrhoea 89
Graafian follicles 8
Granulosa cells 9
Gravida 147
Growth hormone 7
Gumma 100
HAART 98
Haemoglobin 167
HCG 8, 11, 14
Heavy menstrual bleeding 29
HELLP syndrome 174
Herpes 95
Hirsutism causes 47
Hirsutism management 49
HIV 97
Hormone replacement therapy 40
Hormones 6
HPA axis 6
HPV 71
HPV vaccine 75
Human papilloma virus 71
Hyperemesis 144
Hyperprolactinaemia 26
Hypocalvaria 154
Hypothyroidism in pregnancy 152
Hysterosalpingogram 126
Imperforate hymen 68
Implantation 11
In vitro fertilisation 130
Incontinence 59
Induction of labour 195
Infertility 125
Injection 113
Instrumental delivery 208
Insulin resistance 47
Iron infusion 226
Irregular periods 21
Isotretinoin 155
IVF 130
Joel-Cohen incision 214
Kallman syndrome 24
Kleihauer test 159
Koebner phenomenon 65
Krukenberg tumour 78
Labour 18
Lactational mastitis 228

Lactobacilli 83
Lacunae 13
Laparoscopy and dye test 126
Letrozole 49
Leukocytes 166
Levonorgestrel 120
Levonorgestrel coil 117
LH 6
Lichen planus 65
Lichen sclerosus 64
Lichen simplex 65
Listeria 156
Lithium 154
LLETZ 74
Lochia 223
Loop excision 74
Luteal phase 8
Luteinising hormone 6, 15
Lymphogranuloma venereum 88
Macrosomia 162
Magnesium sulfate 195
Marsupialisation 64
Mastitis 228
Maternal sepsis 217
McRoberts manoeuvre 207
Meig's syndrome 53
Melasma 179
Membrane sweep 196
Menarche 7
Menopause 37
Menorrhagia 29
Menstrual cycle 7
Menstruation 8
Metformin 49
Methotrexate 137
Metronidazole 84
Midstream urine 166
Mifepristone 143, 201
Mirabegron 62
Mirena 117
Miscarriage 138
Misoprostol 143, 201
Molar pregnancy 145
Morula 11
Mother and baby unit 228
Mucinous cystadenoma 51
Mucinous retention cysts 56
Mullerian ducts 67
Multiple pregnancy 163
Mycoplasma genitalium 91
Mycoplasma hominis 83
Myomectomy 32
Nabothian cysts 56
Nausea and vomiting 144
NCSP 86
Neonatal abstinence syndrome 154
Nerve injuries 209
Neurosyphilis 101
Nifedipine 195, 202

NIPT 152
Nitrites 165
NSAIDs in pregnancy 153
Nuchal translucency 151
Nucleic acid amplification test 86
Obstetric cholestasis 176
Oestrogen 6, 15
OGTT 48
Oligospermia 128
Onset of labour 192
Ophthalmia neonatorum 91
Oral glucose tolerance test 48
Ovarian cancer 78
Ovarian cysts 50
Ovarian drilling 49, 127
Ovarian hyperstimulation 132
Ovarian torsion 53
Overactive bladder 59
Overflow incontinence 60
Ovulation 10
Ovum 11
Oxytocin 200
Para 147
Partogram 203
Parvovirus B19 157
Patient-controlled analgesia 205
PCOS 46
PE 168
Pelvic exenteration 74
Pelvic inflammatory disease 92
Pelvic organ prolapse 57
Pelvic pain 22
Pemphigoid gestationis 180
Perimenopausal symptoms 38
Perineal massage 211
Perineal tears 209
Pessaries 58
Pethidine 205
Pfannenstiel incision 214
Pipelle biopsy 77
Placenta accreta 185
Placenta increta 185
Placenta percreta 185
Placenta praevia 181
Placental abruption 183
Placental development 12
Placental function 14
Placental growth factor 173
Platelet count 16
Polar body 10
Polycystic ovarian syndrome 46
Polymorphic eruption 179
Post-exposure prophylaxis 100
Postcoital bleeding 22
Postnatal care 223
Postnatal depression 227
Postpartum haemorrhage 212
Postpartum thyroiditis 229
Pre-eclampsia 171

Index

Pregnancy of unknown location 136
Premature labour 193
Premature ovarian insufficiency 39
Premenstrual dysphoric disorder 28
Premenstrual syndrome 27
Preterm 193
Prevotella species 83
Primigravida 147
Primip 147
Primordial follicles 9
Procidentia 58
Progesterone 6, 15, 44
Progestogen implant 115
Progestogen injection 113
Progestogen-only pill 111
Progestogens 44
Prolactin 15, 26
Propess 196
Prostaglandins 18, 201
Prostin 196
Pruritus vulvae 23
Puberty 6
Puerperal psychosis 228
Pulmonary embolism 168
Pyelonephritis 165
Pyogenic granuloma 180
Rapid plasma reagin 101
Rectocele 57
Recurrent miscarriage 140
Red clover 41
Red degeneration of fibroids 33
Remifentanil 205
Retained products 225
Retinopathy screening 175
Retrograde menstruation 33
Rhesus incompatibility 158
Risk of malignancy index 52, 80
Roaccutane 155
Rotterdam criteria 46
RPOC 225
Rubella 155
Rubins manoeuvre 207
Secondary amenorrhoea 26
Secondary follicles 10
Sepsis 217
Septic six 218
Serial growth scans 161
Serous cystadenoma 51
Serous tumours 78
Sex cord-stromal tumours 51, 78
SGA 159
Sheehan's syndrome 231
Shoulder dystocia 207
Sim's speculum 58
Sinusoidal CTG 200
Skin changes in pregnancy 16
Small for gestational age 159
Sodium valproate 154
Spinal anaesthetic 215

Spiral arteries 12
SSRIs 155
Stages of labour 18
Sterilisation 122
Stillbirth 187
Strawberry cervix 94
Stress incontinence 59
Swabs 86
Syncytiotrophoblast 11
Syntocinon 200
Syntometrine 201
Syphilis 100
Tabes dorsalis 101
Tamoxifen 76
Tanner scale 7
Tension-free vaginal tape 62
Teratoma 78
Terbutaline 202
Termination of pregnancy 142
Testosterone (with HRT) 44
Theca folliculi 9
Theca interna 9
Thyroiditis 229
Tibolone 44
Tocolysis 195
Toxoplasmosis 157
Tranexamic acid 202
Transformation zone 55
Treponema pallidum 100
Trichomoniasis 94
Trophoblast 11
Tubal occlusion 122
Twin-twin transfusion 164
Twins 163
UK MEC 104
Ulipristal 120
Umbilical cord 13
Umbilical cord prolapse 206
Urethrocele 57
Urge incontinence 59
Urinary incontinence 59
Urinary tract infection 165
Urine dipstick 165
Urodynamic tests 61
Ursodeoxycholic acid 177
Uterine artery embolisation 32
Uterine artery ligation 213
Uterine dehiscence 220
Uterine hyperstimulation 197
Uterine inversion 221
Uterine prolapse 57
Uterine rupture 220
UTI 165
Vaccines in pregnancy 148
Vaginal agenesis 68
Vaginal birth after caesarean 216
Vaginal discharge 22
Vaginal hypoplasia 68
Vaginal septae 68

Vaginal swabs 86
Variability (CTG) 198
Vasa praevia 182
Vasectomy 122
Vault prolapse 57
VBAC 216
Venous thromboembolism 168
Ventilation-perfusion scan 170
Ventouse 208
VQ scan 170
VTE 168
VTE prophylaxis 169
Vulval cancer 80
Vulval intraepithelial neoplasia 81
Warfarin 154
Wells score 170
Wood's screw manoeuvre 207
Word catheter 64
Yolk sac 12
Zavanelli manoeuvre 207
Zika virus 158
Zygote 11

Printed in Great Britain
by Amazon